UNLOCKING THE DOORS OF DEMENTIA

Practical Help for Families and Their Loved Ones

LAUREN MAHAKIAN

Certified Dementia Practitioner and Elder Care Specialist

outskirts press

Table of Contents

Preface i

*Welcome to My World! * Beyond the Numbers * About Me * What's in This Book*

Section One: The Many Dimensions of Dementia 1

*A History of Dementia * The "Disease" and Its Diagnosis * What's Normal and What's Not * Normal * Not Normal * Alzheimer's Disease * Vascular Dementia * Lewy Body Dementia * Frontotemporal Dementia * Other Forms and Causes of Dementia*

Section Two: The Behaviors of Dementia 15

*First: Step into Their Reality * The Redirection Approach * The Validation Approach*

Confusion and Forgetting 22

Understanding 23

Preventing 24

Responding 25

*Remember That It's Not Personal * Think "Suggest" Instead of "Correct" * Be Brief * Tap into Long-Term Memory * Use "Creative Dementia Talk"*

Anxiety and Agitation 30

Understanding Agitation 30

*Moving * Houseguests * Hospitalization * Changes Related to Caregivers * Home Emergencies * Travel * Threats and Perceived Threats*

Preventing Anxiety 36

*Case the Space * Avoid the Triggers * Monitor Personal Comfort * Simplify Everything*

Responding 38

*Listen to the Frustration * Involve Your Loved One in Activities * Validation and Reassurance * Modify the Environment * Be on Your Best Behavior * Ice Cream * Seek Professional Advice*

Combativeness 42

Understanding 42

Preventing 43

Responding 44

Hallucinations 47

Understanding 47

Responding 48

*Medical Advice * Non-Medical Approaches* 49

Sundowning 50

Understanding 50

Preventing 51

Responding 52

*Keep a Journal * Try Soothing Activities * Timing of Medications * Take Care of Yourself * Ice Cream Therapy*

Suspicions and Delusions 55

Understanding 55

Responding 56

*Remain Calm * Don't Argue * Redirect * Help Others Understand * Replace Valuables * Simplify*

Three-peat (Repeat).. 58

Understanding / Preventing... 58

Responding... 59

*Explore Further * Be Patient and Understanding * Answer the Question * Beyond the Words * Do Something with the Behavior * Develop a New Hobby * Do Something Else * Play Music * Accept It and Move On*

Wandering 62

Understanding... 62

*Disorientation * Confusion * Anxiety * Agitation * Hallucinations * Vision * Warning Signs*

Preventing 64

*Non-Physical Measures * Physical Measures*........................ 65

Responding... 66

Depression 69

Understanding... 69

Responding... 70

Hoarding... 72

Understanding... 72

Responding... 73

*Safety Check * Important Items*

Financial Irresponsibility 76

Understanding 76

Responding 78

Section Three: Handling Difficult Situations 81

Living at Home 84

Understanding 84

Responding 85

Medical Alert System

Moves ("Transitions") 89

Understanding 89

Responding 90

*Planning and Preparing * Where to Move * Making the Transition * After the Transition*

Paying for Daily Care 94

Activities of Daily Living 95

Understanding 95

Responding 96

*Showering * Oral Care * Toileting and Incontinence Care * Medication Management*

Walking, Gait Changes, and Fall Risk 100

Understanding 100

Responding 101

Driving 103

Understanding 103

Responding... 104

    *Continuing to Drive * Taking Away the Keys * Creative
Measures*

Caregiver Guilt.. **110**

  Understanding.. 110

  Responding.. 111

Holidays and Extended Visits............................ **113**

  Understanding.. 113

  Responding.. 114

    Holidays

Sex **117**

  Understanding.. 117

    *Sex and the Person with Dementia * Inappropriate Sexual
Behaviors*

  Responding.. 119

Caring from a Distance **121**

  Understanding.. 122

  Responding.. 122

Palliative Care, Comfort Care, and Hospice **125**

  Understanding.. 125

  Responding.. 126

Closing Thoughts **128**

    *Be Compassionate to Yourself * Talk with Others and Seek
Advice * Get Help*

Preface

Welcome to My World!

Chances are good that you have been touched by someone with dementia. I say that not because you opened this book, but because dementia and Alzheimer's disease affect one in three seniors in the United States. Virtually everyone knows someone involved.

According to facts presented by the Alzheimer's Association (www.alz.org):

- One in three seniors dies with dementia or Alzheimer's. Statistically, an elderly couple is more likely than not to be affected by the disease.
- More than six million Americans live with Alzheimer's disease. Estimates suggest it could rise to as high as 13 million by 2050 as the baby boomer population ages.
- Alzheimer's disease is a leading cause of death in the United States, killing more than breast and prostate cancer combined. While deaths from heart disease are declining (down 14% since 2000), deaths from Alzheimer's disease have more than doubled.

But you did open this book, so you are probably looking for answers to difficult questions about dementia or are searching for solutions to challenging situations or behaviors you are unprepared to handle. You are not alone. Across the United States, family caregivers are under tremendous stress from caring for their loved ones with dementia.

Again turning to the Alzheimer's Association, they report:

- Eleven million Americans provide unpaid care for people with dementia, totaling 18 billion hours in 2022.
- Family caregivers for people with dementia are nearly twice as likely to report that their health has gotten worse due to care responsibilities than family caregivers for older people without dementia (35% versus 19%).

Beyond the Numbers

That may be dementia by the numbers, but numbers don't tell the story of the affected person who fears losing their independence. They don't help relieve the frustration and stress of the family who struggles to provide care. They don't help make ends meet when finances get stretched thin as care costs rise. They don't address the difficulties faced by medical professionals who are powerless to change the course of the disease. Medical professionals are often reluctant to inform patients of a diagnosis because there is no cure.

About Me

As a care manager to the chronologically gifted for over fifteen years, I see dozens of people with dementia daily. I help their caregivers and families reduce stress by offering solutions to the challenges presented by the many dimensions of dementia. I've seen countless challenging behaviors and stressful situations, from the guy who only ate hot dogs, peanuts, and potato chips, to the woman who battled anyone trying to help her even though she couldn't remember the last time she ate.

It isn't easy caring for your aging loved one. It's even more stressful with dementia, with or without a formal diagnosis. Forgetting to pay bills or not remembering your visit yesterday is frustrating to address.

Changes in how your loved one acts and behaves are even more challenging. Dementia is not just a memory decline. In many ways, your loved one becomes different from the one you've known your whole life. Your relationship may have to change in fundamental ways. If you don't change your approach, you will get frustrated and stressed, and your health will suffer. You need help.

I wrote this book to answer many commonly asked questions and offer advice on confronting the challenges of caring for a loved one with memory impairment and its accompanying behaviors.

What's in This Book

I designed this book for anyone caring for someone exhibiting symptoms of dementia. I'll try to use the term "loved one" to refer to the person with dementia, as that term certainly fits. Whether it is your parent, sibling, spouse, or another family member, it is an act of true love to provide or oversee care for someone suffering from these many dimensions of dementia.

There are many online resources and other books to learn about dementia and its diagnosis. They can be overwhelming and confusing. Not all discussions will fit your situation, and — especially without a formal diagnosis — you may struggle to match the symptoms you see with those attributed to various dementias.

Much of what I discuss in this book involves behaviors associated with dementia and does not require a formal diagnosis. As I often say, I am not a doctor, I don't want to be a doctor, and I do not dispense medical advice. But as someone who has been actively dealing with dementia professionally for over a decade, helping hundreds of families reduce their stress, I've seen a thing or two. Hopefully, sharing those experiences can help with your situation.

I didn't write this book to describe dementia or its diagnosis, but we still need to start there. We'll try to maintain a practical perspective of someone helping families daily to help to establish a common baseline for further conversation. We can then discuss specific approaches to many stressful situations you may encounter. I'll try to avoid medical jargon and instead focus on its meaning, using medical terms when appropriate. I may cite a few references, but most of the content comes from my over fifteen years of experience working with the chronologically gifted.

This book has three sections.

- **The Many Dimensions of Dementia** section summarizes the condition and discusses the nature of Alzheimer's disease and other specific dementias. It's intended to offer insight into the heart of each from a non-medical, practical perspective—their diagnosis, underlying causes, and common symptoms and behaviors.
- **The Behaviors of Dementia** section addresses many common behaviors you may face, with or without a formal diagnosis of dementia. Many behaviors can appear, and we need to prepare for them. We will seek to understand each identified behavior, learn how to prevent it, and discuss how to respond when it does occur.
- The **Handling Difficult Situations** section offers my tips and suggestions for handling the many everyday situations caregivers find themselves in. Here we tackle potentially stressful issues such as how to take away the car, survive holidays with family, caregiving from a distance, and the guilt you may experience when making difficult decisions. We will also discuss suggestions for successful visits, understanding end-of-life care, and more.

Throughout the book, you will also learn about practical approaches to interacting with your loved one in new ways, using effective techniques such as redirection and validation. My goal is to help significantly reduce the stress caused by caring for your loved one with dementia. It's not an easy job.

Let's get started.

SECTION ONE
THE MANY DIMENSIONS OF DEMENTIA

DEMENTIA IS A general term that describes someone with memory impairment. Despite growing awareness, it often presents initially as somewhat puzzling when you face it with a family member. Often, conversations include:

- "Come on, Mom. Don't you recognize your grandkids?"
- "Your keys? They're attached to your purse, so you don't lose them, remember?"
- "Dad, you said that just a few minutes ago. Don't you think I heard you?"

Most people are unprepared for a decline in their loved ones. They are slow to recognize it and ill-equipped to address the situation positively, which can affect the quality of life and happiness of the person with the condition. Worse, perhaps, is the frustration and stress that grows in loved ones caring for them, leading to a general decline in the well-being of everyone connected to the disease.

Alzheimer's disease is also gaining awareness, but most people believe that Alzheimer's disease and dementia are the same. Let's begin by distinguishing between the two to start in the right direction.

Alzheimer's disease is a disease of the brain. It is irreversible and progressive. There are underlying medical causes that continue to be aggressively studied, looking for ways to prevent them.

Dementia is not a specific disease. Instead, it represents a variety of symptoms commonly accompanied by declining memory. Presenting with dementia is symptomatic of Alzheimer's disease.

While Alzheimer's disease accounts for more than half of all diagnosed cases of dementia, dementia can also result from other underlying conditions, including Parkinson's disease and Huntington's disease. Frontotemporal dementia results from progressive degeneration of the temporal and frontal lobes of the brain. Lewy body dementia is a disease where abnormal deposits of a protein affect chemicals in the brain. Vascular dementia results from insufficient blood flow to the brain due to narrowing or blocked blood vessels, which can arise from stroke, diabetes, high cholesterol, or other conditions. In mixed dementia or "other" dementias, the underlying cause may be less clear.

It is also vital for those caring for someone with dementia to understand that declining memory is not the only symptom. **The Behaviors of Dementia** section of this book offers an overview of many others. Failing to realize that these behaviors result from severe changes in the brain can cause frustration, anxiety, conflict, anger, and even family drama.

Whatever the cause of a person's dementia, families must also understand that it is progressive and irreversible, resulting in worsening dementia over time. Symptoms may be controlled or slowed with medication, but ineffectively. Understanding how to manage care for those with dementia can help and is the purpose of this book.

A History of Dementia

It wasn't that long ago that the term "dementia" was not widely used. Great Uncle Ned was "senile" for his forgetfulness. Aunt Sally was "eccentric" for her quirky behaviors. Despite being first used to describe the most noticeable symptoms of dementia in 1797, the term initially referred to someone with a mental deficiency. Later, it came to refer to someone who had lost the ability to reason or function psychologically and socially, including from curable conditions.

Dementia, however, is far from a new occurrence and may date to prehistoric times. Ancient literature discusses a dementia-like condition resulting from old age, which few achieved. The Greek philosopher Pythagoras divided the human lifespan into phases, the final described as a period of mental and physical decay until "The mind is reduced to the imbecility of the first epoch of infancy." Seven Byzantine emperors who had reached the age of 70 showed signs of dementia.

Until the industrial era, dementia was relatively rare, likely because it most commonly affects people over 80. Such lifespans were uncommon in preindustrial times. Still, dementia caused by disease was known, presenting as a mental illness caused by brain-destroying diseases like syphilis. Syphilitic dementia was widespread until the use of penicillin after WWII.

Only in recent history has medical science helped us to understand that dementia is not a normal function of aging but rather a result of several underlying causes.

The "Disease" and Its Diagnosis

Throughout this book, I will remind you periodically that I am not a doctor and do not wish to be a doctor. I do not offer medical advice and try to avoid medical jargon. Instead, I want to focus on the nature of dementia and what you, the caregiver, can do to help your loved one and yourself.

I'll refer to dementia as "the disease," whether classified as a disease (like Alzheimer's) or not. It may be scientifically inaccurate, but accuracy would add confusion.

I will also refer to the stages of dementia or cognitive impairment. These stages mainly refer to the progression of Alzheimer's disease, but they are gauged based on the symptoms and degree of cognitive impairment. I have found it helpful to use the same descriptive terms to refer to stages of dementia in general. Those stages are:

- No Cognitive Impairment
- Mild Cognitive Impairment
- Moderate Cognitive Impairment
- Severe Cognitive Impairment
- Very Severe Cognitive Impairment or Vegetative

These stages of Alzheimer's are not even well agreed to in medical literature. Some practitioners include as few as three stages, while others may consist of as many as ten. Seven is common, but including more than five doesn't improve our understanding. Assessing a person for dementia follows loosely defined guidelines. A professional may deem a person as having mild symptoms in some areas while moderate or severe in others. It's not an exact science, so finer granularity doesn't help much.

The Montreal Cognitive Assessment, or MoCA, attempts to more objectively quantify the level of cognitive impairment using a 30-point scale based on a test instrument, evaluating various aspects of memory such as recall, attention, and language. While it is technically an objective test, even this may not accurately reflect the severity of a person's dementia or match other behaviors exhibited.

I'm frequently asked about medical exams to diagnose the underlying disease. All dementias are diagnosed based on symptoms and health history, although medical imaging may rule out other causes. Also, medical evaluation does not always result in an accurate diagnosis. Lewy body dementia can appear as Parkinson's disease, and Lewy bodies can occur in Parkinson's. Amyloid plaque accumulation in the brain accompanies Alzheimer's, but such plaques can exist without developing Alzheimer's symptoms. Only after death can an autopsy reveal the actual cause.

The important things to remember about the disease and its symptoms are:

- It won't get better
- It can't be cured or reversed
- It will likely get worse

What's Normal and What's Not

Since most dementias are evaluated subjectively, based on symptoms and often a level of cognitive impairment, it's helpful to know what's normal and what's not.

NORMAL

You've likely been in a room in your home, realized you needed something from another room, and walked there to retrieve that item—only to forget what you were looking for. Have you searched for a set of keys, a checkbook, or a purse? They're always in the last place you look, right?

Losing or forgetting minor things is normal when busy or preoccupied. Also, don't confuse someone forgetting with them not listening. We believe we're listening, but we're not paying close attention. Asked what you just heard, you may not be able to recall.

It's normal to lose items or forget where we last left something occasionally. Usually, something triggers just before we locate it. We forget things that are easily forgettable when thinking about other matters, even if those things are important to remember, like where we parked the car at the mall.

NOT NORMAL

However, forgetting important things and people in your life is not normal. The names of your grandchildren. Memories, like your wedding or the birth of your children. People who work a regular schedule quickly recall the day of the week. Retired persons often don't, but they can reason it out based on other events.

Below is a rough guide to normal "forgetting" and signs of possible memory impairment. The contrast between "normal" and "suspect" is deliberate. In the earliest stages of dementia, the shift from the first column to the second is gradual. In the end, the last item sums it up nicely. You're probably okay if you're worried about your memory while others are not.

	Normal	Suspect
Events	Occasionally forget details of events. Unable to recall details of a conversation from a month or two ago.	Frequently forget details of even recent events. Unable to recall details of a conversation of just days or weeks ago.
Names	Not remembering the name of an acquaintance or someone you just met, even moments ago.	Not remembering the names of family members. Not recognizing family members even if their appearance has not changed since last seeing them.
Language	Occasionally having difficulty finding the right word while speaking.	Frequently struggle to find words, substituting words for others.
Memory	You worry about your memory. Your close friends and relatives do not.	Your close friends and relatives are worried about your memory. You may be aware of problems but think it's normal and begin using coping mechanisms.

Of course, our challenge is recognizing cognitive impairments in our loved ones. If you suspect dementia, get your loved one to a physician for an evaluation. Be advised, however, that a 2015 study by the Alzheimer's Association found that physicians are often reluctant to inform patients of a dementia diagnosis. The disclosure rate was 45% for Alzheimer's diagnosis and a shockingly low 27% for other dementias. The reasons for this low disclosure rate are unclear but seem to be improving in the last few years. The report cited fear of causing emotional distress, which may also be related to a medical inability to reverse or cure the disease.

If you suspect dementia, begin immediately preparing for the later stages of the disease. See the chapters in **Handling Difficult Situations** for advice on health and finance. If your loved one is diagnosed with significant cognitive impairment, they can no longer make critical financial decisions.

Coping mechanisms can be helpful to someone showing early signs of dementia. Being organized and practicing habitual behaviors and routines helps a lot. Establish a place for keys, wallets or purses, checkbooks, bank cards, etc., and replace them there.

At the same time, however, when your loved one uses coping mechanisms to mask early warning signs of her memory impairment, it makes it that much more difficult for you to recognize her impairment and seek help. Open dialogue and a non-judgmental attitude are helpful.

Alzheimer's Disease

Alzheimer's disease is the leading cause of dementia, affecting more than 5 million people in the United States. It typically has onset in the mid-sixties, although "early-onset" Alzheimer's accounts for less than 10% of diagnoses.

The causes of Alzheimer's disease are not well understood, but it damages and kills brain cells, which causes a progressive decline in memory and mental function, as well as personality changes and many of the behaviors discussed in this book.

The most common risk factor for developing Alzheimer's is growing old, but it is important to note that it is a disease and not a normal part of aging. There is also some evidence that lifestyle and health are risk factors. Other studies indicate that lifelong learning and social engagement may reduce the risk of developing Alzheimer's. Conversely, low education and isolation may increase risk. There is also evidence of genetic predisposition for Alzheimer's. Studies are ongoing in this area.

There are unmistakable hallmarks of the disease in the brain. One is the accumulation of amyloid plaque, clumps of a protein called beta-amyloid, which may cause the death of brain cells. The other hallmark is the presence of "tangles," abnormally twisted threads of another protein called tau, causing a disruption to the regular transport of nutrients and materials that may also cause the death of brain cells.

Alzheimer's disease and its symptoms worsen over time. Some treatments may slow symptom progression, but there is no cure.

Vascular Dementia

Vascular dementia is another common dementia, second only to Alzheimer's disease. Diagnosis can be challenging, so good estimates for the number of people afflicted with the disease are unavailable. Still, it accounts for just under 20% of dementia in older adults. It has many of the common symptoms of dementia, including memory loss and wandering, but adds hallucinations and delusions. A person with vascular dementia may begin to experience balance and coordination issues, laugh at inappropriate times (such as the misfortune of others), or have difficulty controlling their bladder or bowel.

Unlike most other dementias, symptoms often appear suddenly rather than developing slowly over time. If there is any suspicion of vascular dementia, such as after a stroke, or if your loved one has any risk factors (high blood pressure, high cholesterol, smoking, atherosclerosis, diabetes, obesity), seek medical attention immediately. An early diagnosis may minimize the impact.

Following a stroke, vascular dementia may onset, which significantly guides its diagnosis.

Note that a person with Alzheimer's can also experience vascular dementia. Complicating diagnosis in some cases, the symptoms of vascular dementia may appear gradually, as they do in Alzheimer's disease.

Lewy Body Dementia

Lewy body dementia, or LBD, is another common cause of dementia, behind Alzheimer's disease and vascular dementia. LBD is a disease resulting from deposits of the protein alpha-synuclein in the brain. These deposits are Lewy bodies and affect chemicals that control mood, thinking, and behavior.

In perhaps the most high-profile case, actor-comedian Robin Williams became overwhelmed by paranoia and was so confused he couldn't remember any lines while making a film. He was diagnosed with Parkinson's disease just months before his death by suicide in 2014, but his autopsy revealed that he had Lewy body dementia.

LBD affects over a million people in the United States. It typically onsets after age fifty but has been seen in younger people. In addition to memory loss and confusion, those with LBD experience changes in thinking, delusions, and visual hallucinations. Those affected can have difficulty interpreting what they see into information and can exhibit symptoms like Parkinson's disease, including balance issues, rigidity, and hunched posture.

The symptoms of LBD may vary with the affected parts of the brain. Lewy bodies may deposit in nerve cells in the brain regions involved in emotions, behaviors, sleep, thinking, language, perception, memory, the senses, and movement.

As with other dementias, LBD progresses with time. Life expectancy from diagnosis to death is five to seven years but can vary from two to 20 years. How quickly symptoms develop varies greatly from person to person, depending on overall health, age, and severity of symptoms.

LBD can be very similar to Alzheimer's disease in its early stages. LBD is also commonly associated with Parkinson's disease. LBD can occur with or without Parkinson's disease.

Frontotemporal Dementia

Frontotemporal dementia, which I've heard called frontal lobe dementia by some doctors, can be caused by several disorders that affect both the frontal and temporal lobes of the brain, resulting in their atrophy or shrinkage. These are brain areas associated with personality, behavior, decision-making, language, and movement.

Not surprisingly, a common characteristic of frontotemporal dementia is a dramatic personality change. Behavior, as well as interpersonal relationships, can also change significantly. Frontotemporal dementia can onset much earlier than Alzheimer's, affecting people in their 50s and 60s. It sometimes afflicts people in their 20s or as late as their 80s.

There are many forms of frontotemporal dementia, characterized primarily by behavioral changes, language disturbances, or muscle complications. It may be mistaken for a psychiatric problem or early-onset Alzheimer's disease.

Behavioral variant frontotemporal dementia results in dramatic personality changes, including loss of empathy or developing apathy. Compulsive behaviors may surface, along with inappropriate behaviors or poor judgment. Changes in eating habits are also common, often overeating but sometimes eating less. You may also notice changes in personal hygiene. In many cases, the person developing this form of dementia is unaware of the changes in their behaviors.

Primary progressive aphasia affects language skills like speaking, writing, and understanding. Sometimes, a person may become unable to form sentences (semantic aphasia). In other cases, a person's speech becomes labored and lacks grammar skills they once had (nonfluent/agrammatic aphasia).

Frontotemporal dementia can also affect motor functions, such as in ALS (Amyotrophic Lateral Sclerosis, or Lou Gehrig's disease). Limbs can become stiff and uncoordinated, such as in corticobasal syndrome. Progressive supranuclear palsy causes muscle stiffness, changes in posture, difficulty walking, or eye movement.

All forms of frontotemporal dementia affect the ability to think, reason, and function. If your loved one has been diagnosed with frontotemporal dementia, they will likely become increasingly dependent on caregivers for activities of daily living. The progression of the disease and expected lifespans vary greatly.

Other Forms and Causes of Dementia

Several other conditions can lead to dementia. I won't detail the differences here, mainly because symptoms of dementia are widely varied in the first place. Discuss the diagnosis and prognosis with your loved one's physician and learn as much as possible about the disease. Some advice in this book under **The Behaviors of Dementia** may greatly help when negative behaviors result.

Parkinson's disease is a neurodegenerative disorder that affects neurons that produce dopamine in the brain. Tremors, slow movement, rigidity, and balance problems can result.

Huntington's disease is a genetic disorder that breaks down nerve cells in the brain. As the disease progresses, physical and mental abilities continue to decline.

Mixed dementia is a condition where multiple types of dementia or several underlying causes coincide. It's common for a person to suffer from Alzheimer's and other forms of dementia, for example.

Alcohol dementia, as implied, results from excessive alcohol abuse over time. The resulting neurological damage results in a global loss of cognitive function with many symptoms. In effect, a "mixed dementia," Alcohol dementia has many of the symptoms of frontotemporal dementia.

I'll close this **The Many Dimensions of Dementia** section with a reminder that dementia is diagnosed almost entirely based on symptoms, commonly including a decline in short-term memory function. I, therefore, leave on the table one last cause of dementia — "other." Only after an autopsy can science hope to understand the cause of a person's dementia.

Now let's get on with the heart of this book: what can you expect, and what can you do about it?

SECTION TWO

The Behaviors of Dementia

IN MY WORK as a care manager to the chronologically gifted, the most common phone call I get from a prospective client involves some new behavior that Mom started "suddenly," and they don't know what to do about it. More typically, forgetfulness, confusion, or anxiety were present for a while and only recently led to uncomfortable situations. While you were busy with your life, it was easy to miss her slow changes that suddenly make sense when confronted by an outburst or episode of confusion.

- Mom abandoned her old car after it overheated, relying on total strangers to return home, and then had no recollection of where she'd left her vehicle.
- Family members visit Dad for the first time in years and are shocked by his sudden memory decline or his combativeness.
- Aunt Sally didn't return for hours when grocery shopping, wandering without purpose.

These are just a few of the calls I've gotten over more than a decade. I'm the one that people call when they don't know where to turn. I help families negotiate the turbulent and unpredictable waters of dementia.

The behaviors I present in this section are some I encounter most often in my practice. For each, I'll describe the behavior, address how to prevent it, and end with suggestions.

I should acknowledge that some behaviors result from an underlying condition. Once we address that condition, the behavior may disappear. Those are the easy ones.

Most aberrant behaviors are chronic or sporadic. They may hide for a long time until triggered for a reason that escapes us. Their underlying condition is dementia, for which there is no cure.

Although we can't eliminate these behavioral challenges, we can use well-established techniques to mitigate them. The trick is not to respond instinctively, but instead work to understand them and respond with an appropriate approach.

Fortunately, two approaches, **Redirection** and **Validation**, often work for various behaviors.

First: Step into Their Reality

Both redirection and validation are rooted in empathy for your loved one. That empathy only comes by putting yourself in your loved one's shoes. Consider their reality and imagine yourself in their situation.

For example, Mom may not remember the day of the week or recognize a photo of her grandchildren. Maybe she remembers her husband but not the faces or names of one or more of her children. After a career, she may imagine herself still working as CEO of a company or as an airline pilot. I've seen it all. I try to imagine her life before dementia – how she interacted with others, what she did most days, what hobbies she enjoyed, and more. Losing those aspects of her life has emotional consequences. Understanding the past may produce clues about where the behaviors are rooted.

The Redirection Approach

Redirection is a technique that, to the uninitiated, may seem unfair or show a lack of respect for the loved one with dementia. The opposite is the case. It is a tried-and-true technique to shift focus away from a situation that results in annoying or unsafe behavior to bring calm. The result is that everyone, including your loved one, is happier. Your loved one moves on to something that brings comfort or distracts attention from the situation that caused distress. The approach enhances, not diminishes, dignity and respect.

UNDERSTANDING

Recall that dementia is not just about losing memory. It is a complex condition that presents in many ways, and often those ways include undesirable behaviors. Dad may repeatedly say, in an agitated state, "I want to go home. I want to go home!" Reason and logic have failed, and the statement has little to do with an actual place and more to do with wanting comfort. While this often happens after a move to a new living situation, it also occurs with people with dementia in their own homes.

Typical responses to negative behaviors confront what they appear to be. For example, in the case of the agitated person repeating, "I want to go home," a typical and inappropriate response is, "You can't go home," "You are home," or, worse, "But we sold your home!" These responses do not address the underlying issue, which likely has nothing to do with home.

Redirecting your loved one from that state of mind is in everyone's best interest. We must address negative behaviors, especially those that cause harm or stress.

Perhaps the best thing about redirection is that it often works even while you struggle to understand the underlying issue.

RESPONDING

Redirection is not hard to use once you emotionally detach from the situation and can control your emotions to act confidently in a leadership capacity. Leadership is what's needed. Your loved one needs to follow a new direction, shifting focus from whatever is causing the behavior.

Redirection fails when the caregiver isn't confident in what they're trying to accomplish and why it's essential. Lack of confidence is usually due to emotional attachment and not understanding the underlying issue.

Therefore, I recommend that any caregiver begin with empathy. Understand that your loved one isn't behaving the way they are entirely by choice. Acknowledge their feelings. Telling them that they are wrong will immediately set up confrontation and mistrust.

Once you acknowledge there is something behind the behavior at hand, you are in a position to ask questions that can provide additional insight. My favorite line of questioning follows this general progression:

- Are you hungry?
- Are you thirsty?
- Do you want to change something?

Once we eliminate the first two possible issues, the third question usually leads to understanding the source of the behavior. You probably know your loved one better than anyone, so use your instinct to explore underlying causes. A few non-judgmental questions that may help include:

- Do you need to go to the bathroom?
- Are you uncomfortable sitting here?
- Do you want to go to a different room?
- Are you tired? (or hot or cold; address their physical needs)
- Can I bring you something?

You can also use open-ended questions, such as:

- Tell me what's bothering you.

- How can I help you?
- What would you like to change/do right now?

Leading with empathy and more information than you originally had, you can now redirect your loved one better.

You will then use the responses to shift focus from the current situation to a new, desired one. "I understand, Mom. Why don't we join this activity over here?" Or something like, "I remember you made the most amazing breakfasts. The smells were incredible. Do you smell baking in the kitchen? Let's go check it out." There are also many ways to take advantage of the current surroundings, simply bridging from something in the environment to a new activity. "Wow, it's a gorgeous day! Should we take a short walk and look at the plants?"

Redirection, done well, can offer relief for even the most dangerous or troublesome behaviors while preserving the dignity and well-being of your loved one.

The Validation Approach

Validation is another technique to help better understand your loved one and address their behaviors. At first glance, validation seems like redirection and uses some of the same methods. It is also rooted in empathy and understanding your loved one and the causes of their behavior.

The validation approach accepts your loved one for who they are at this moment in time and seeks to validate the feelings, however distorted. Rather than ignoring false realities, it validates the feelings and emotions your loved one is experiencing, which is their reality. Often, validation looks to understand what issues from the past your loved one may be resolving, looking for closure after keeping feelings hidden for a very long time.

Confusion and Forgetting

Memory loss and confusion are possibly the most widely recognized symptoms of dementia. In fact, following its introduction in 1797, the term "dementia" became synonymous with declining memory by the early 20th century.

Despite widespread awareness of dementia and memory loss, it can be challenging to identify, especially if you see your loved one frequently. Slow changes seem normal, but, later, as the disease progresses, they become incredibly difficult to deal with.

We all forget things. I'd swear I left my glasses on the table in the living room but found them on my nightstand. My friend is always looking for his keys or his wallet. We see a familiar person in the checkout line at the grocery store but can't recall their name. Have you ever purposefully walked into a room only to then forget why?

These are everyday "forgetting" events, not necessarily signs of declining memory. How many different places did my friend place his keys last year? Is it unreasonable to expect him to remember precisely where he left them the very last time? Of course not. He might then recall that his routine was interrupted and walk directly to where the keys are hiding, or he might find the keys and then remember how they got there.

The fact that we all forget things occasionally makes it challenging to distinguish the signs of abnormal memory decline and diagnose dementia in its early stages. Even more confounding is that habits—behaviors, rituals, and often-repeated complex tasks (such as driving)—can mask an abnormal memory decline for years. "Mom went to church every Sunday. She called me every Wednesday at 6:00 PM. She got together with her neighbors every afternoon at 4 o'clock. Why can't she remember the names of my children?"

Understanding

The primary underlying cause of memory loss and confusion is the progressive damage to brain cells. While it's well-documented for Alzheimer's, virtually all dementias worsen. Symptoms that are initially mild become more pronounced as time passes.

Memory loss and confusion may be very mild in the early stages and difficult to recognize in your loved one. He may be aware of the changes in his ability to recall things he knows he should, such as your children's names or what to call that kitchen utensil. He might not remember even recent events and have difficulty making decisions. He may have trouble understanding what you're telling him. These situations may frustrate him, triggering other behaviors discussed later in this book.

Your loved one may begin to use memory devices to mitigate their impairment. These devices are not inherently wrong but can mask the extent of their memory impairment. From attaching keys to her purse so she can't misplace them to posting sticky notes with grandchildren's names near the phone, this "masking" behavior is typical in the early stages of dementia. Unfortunately, it can also conceal the extent of memory impairment for years.

Memory loss becomes more severe in the later stages of the disease. Your loved one may completely forget your children's names or fail to recognize family members. Shown photographs of even immediate family members, he may ask, "Who's that?" He may forget his wife's name but still know she is someone special to him. Looking at a spoon, he may refer to it as a fork or use any words to substitute for another term he can't readily recall.

Time confusion is another symptom of severe memory impairment. Your loved one may complain that you never visit her, even though you saw her only yesterday. She may not know the current month, year, or season. Taking her away from home, she may soon ask if it's time to go home, unaware it's been just a few minutes. She may forget the purpose of everyday items, such as a pen or a fork. These changes are some of the most painful for caregivers and families.

Confusion is common when sleep is interrupted, such as needing to use the toilet. Disorientation from the dark may contribute to the confusion, and some believe it's morning or say they need to go to work (even though they stopped working many years ago). Others no longer notice the difference between night and day. In extreme cases, some people with dementia experience a complete reversal of their normal sleep pattern, staying up all night, and then sleeping all day. If your loved one exhibits confusion, consider poor sleep may be a contributing factor.

In general, declining memory is very frustrating for your loved one, just as it may frustrate you. However, you can rationalize your frustration and learn ways to cope. Your loved one can't, which can lead to more frustration, confusion, anxiety, and any of the other behaviors discussed in this book.

Preventing

Science continues to look for ways to prevent or reduce damage to brain cells and resulting memory loss. Unfortunately, no current medication succeeds at this, although they may reduce symptoms for a while.

Although we can't reverse memory loss, there are devices we can use to help loved ones be less confused in the early stages of the disease. Many of the masking techniques described above can also help. Eliminating trips away from home also helps since any trip can trigger confusion and lead to an unexpected situation.

Try to keep conversations simple. Avoiding complex topics, such as current events or politics, can help eliminate stress and confusion. Speaking of recent events, turn off television news! It's filled with scary stories and adds stress to many with dementia, not to mention it adds confusion. Instead, watch shows that aren't upsetting or, better yet, turn on music your loved one enjoys.

Generally speaking, find ways to create routines. Ritual behaviors help reduce confusion. Add labels to cupboards and drawers, for example. Sticking to a daily schedule can also help. All of this helps avoid unnecessary confusion for someone with dementia.

Responding

In the early stages of dementia, you may not recognize the symptoms. If your loved one struggles with a word or name, try not to quickly complete her sentences, which is easy to do in our haste to move on to other topics or tasks. Instead, explore the extent of memory impairment and see if she can remember without your help. Avoid criticism, which is all too easy to offer. "Come on, Mom. That's Sally, don't you remember?"

Especially if your loved one lives independently, don't show alarm or say anything threatening his independence. He will undoubtedly begin masking his memory loss to conceal the true extent of his impairment.

As the disease progresses, memory loss can manifest in many ways. Don't point out if your loved one doesn't remember a name. Instead, find ways to avoid her needing to remember names. If someone is visiting, introduce them, even if Mom remembers. If your loved one refers to a stranger as a "neighbor," let her. Find ways to "just go with it."

Here are a few simple tips that may help:

REMEMBER THAT IT'S NOT PERSONAL

Remember that the disease is causing your loved one not to remember important things. All memory is affected, not just unimportant memories from the past. It's not personal if they call you by the wrong name or don't recognize you. Don't show negative emotion. Becoming upset doesn't help your loved one. It just hurts you and adds to their confusion.

THINK "SUGGEST" INSTEAD OF "CORRECT"

When your loved one uses a wrong word or name, don't correct her. Too often, I hear my clients talking harshly to their loved ones out of frustration. Instead of, "Mom, that's not Pam. That's Paula!" try, "I think that's Paula, right?" It may be difficult at first, but it becomes second nature with time and can significantly enhance your enjoyment of her as her memory impairment progresses.

BE BRIEF

Long explanations or reasoning are useless to your loved one and can be overwhelming. Be as brief as possible and be transparent. Don't offer choices. Instead, tell them what you will do and ask if that's okay.

TAP INTO LONG-TERM MEMORY

Long-term memory often remains when other memories fade. **Photographs** or items with sentimental value can trigger long-term memory of people, places, and things. For example, a person with significant memory loss may not recognize someone today, even if they are in the room, but they may recognize them from a photo taken thirty or forty years ago. The photos may evoke more memories leading to loved ones recalling good times or describing events in detail that we've long forgotten. Photos are a great way to turn an uncomfortable situation with an old friend or relative into a positive one.

Music also is compelling for tapping into long-term memory. We've all had an experience where we hear a song playing and instantly recall an important event from long ago. We may not know why we are suddenly transported to another place and time, but we understand it relates to our long-term memory, where we tuck meaningful memories that we don't use often. The same is often true of our loved ones with dementia.

Music has long been known to be a great help in caring for those with memory impairments. The film *Alive Inside* focuses on the remarkable ability of music to "awaken the soul" of people, some with advanced dementia or Alzheimer's disease.

Try using popular songs during your loved one's formative years to tap into long-term memory. If you see no reaction, try popular music from their late teens and early twenties. If you don't get a positive response, try another music genre from the same period.

One of the most rewarding activities for stimulating long-term memory involves something simple: **facial care and makeup**. I say rewarding because the emotional response from many people (often, but not exclusively, women) is an instant connection to another place and time.

Many women routinely wore makeup in their younger years. Over time, they gradually slowed, increasingly reserving their use of makeup for special occasions. Now faced with dementia, there aren't many special occasions to look forward to.

As an activity for those in the early stages of dementia, we focus primarily on stimulation and a sense of purpose. What better way to connect with your loved one than to get ready for an outing? First, participants can enjoy the anticipation of a scenic drive or even a stop for ice cream. The sense of purpose comes from their role in the activity: getting ready.

Even men and women who never (or rarely) used makeup can enjoy the build-up to an outing and the stimulation of getting prepared. The activity includes selecting clothing, washing, shaving, dressing, and focusing on personal appearance. Sit with your loved one and help them prepare, whether applying makeup or giving advice on what to wear. A new article of clothing, or a soothing hand massage, might add just the right touch.

Working on their physical appearance empowers our loved ones; a little pampering can do a world of good.

For those in the later stages of the disease, the same activity can evoke long-forgotten memories. I've seen women light up, seeing themselves in the mirror with lipstick for the first time in years. Who doesn't smile seeing Dad looking dapper as he poses proudly in front of the mirror? Make sure you have plenty of time and be prepared to hear stories from long ago. As I like to say, "Just roll with it!" You never want to lose the opportunity to connect with your loved one's long-term memory.

Self-care and pampering, with or without makeup, are easy to do with your loved one and require minimal planning. Combining them with a simple planned activity adds an essential sense of purpose for those in many stages of the disease. This helps to boost self-confidence and also pass the time productively.

Other techniques to tap into long-term memory include watching classic films that may trigger a response, or painting on a blank canvas. You may be surprised by what your loved one creates.

USE "CREATIVE DEMENTIA TALK"

There are several ways to communicate through dementia, but first, you must accept that your loved one will never be how you remember or want. Especially with time confusion, they may take you on remarkable journeys if you follow them rather than correct them with facts. Remember, this is their reality. Step into that reality and have fun. It's much more rewarding than stressing out about what you can't change.

Marjorie lived in a memory care facility with her husband of more than sixty years. Although they lived in separate rooms, they spent much time together in common areas with many others.

As I sat with the pair, Marjorie could not tell me the name of the man seated next to her or identify him as her husband. She did understand that he was somehow important to her, holding her hand over her heart. She also failed to recognize current photos of her three sons.

Her face lit up when shown old photos of her boys as children. She began chatting about the mischief they used to get into. She teared up when shown a photo of her wedding and smiled seeing photos of the two of them together more than thirty years ago.

Long-term memory is often very much intact after short-term memory fails. Photographs, like music, can tap into this long-term memory and create positive experiences.

Anxiety and Agitation

Agitation and anxiety are widespread in those who have dementia. We'll address both since one often leads to the other.

Before we start, I must emphasize that anyone experiencing abnormal behavioral symptoms must seek medical attention and receive a thorough medical check-up. Medical professionals may identify underlying causes, especially when abnormal behaviors appear suddenly. Treatment of an underlying condition depends on accurate diagnosis and exploring possible causes and the behaviors the person is experiencing.

Some of the reasons I've seen corrected quickly include:

- Diet and nutrition
- Medical condition (possibly undiagnosed)
- Medications or interaction between medications

In addition to arising from an underlying condition, agitation and anxiety are common symptoms of dementia. They also can lead to other behaviors addressed in this book. In these cases, the sufferer is experiencing biological changes that significantly impede his ability to handle and process new information, confront new challenges, and negotiate new stimuli the way he did in the past. It is a direct result of the disease.

Understanding Agitation

We need a two-pronged approach to anxiety and agitation. First, we avoid situations we know will trigger them. Then, when they do occur, we need to respond effectively and restore calm.

Anxiety and agitation often exist in those with dementia because their world changes as the disease progresses. Daily life is increasingly challenging, and disruptions are confusing, which can be scary and exhausting for your loved one.

Anxiety is often suppressed or masked, hidden beneath the surface, until triggered. The most common trigger is a change to daily routine, planned or unplanned. Remember that your loved one is most comfortable in the practices they developed over time. These routines provide a framework for daily activities, from preparing and eating meals to bathing. Anything that disrupts these routines can trigger episodes of anxiety or even extreme agitation.

To understand where this behavior comes from, try objectively looking at their experiences and environment. They may be feeling isolated, ignored, or misunderstood. They may be experiencing changes in their environment or unable to make sense of their surrounds, which could make them feel confused or unsafe. They may even be dealing with physical frustrations like pain, feeling hot or cold, hunger, or thirst.

These frustrations come down to a lack of control over the situation and are compounded even further by not being able to communicate one's needs.

Let's look at a few common triggers.

MOVING

Moving is stressful for most of us, even without dementia. For those with dementia, a move is even more stressful because it shatters comfortable routines and demands new ones. It may be permanent, such as transitioning to a memory care community or nursing home. It may also be temporary, such as a hospital stay.

Plan any move to mitigate stress. Help ensure the smoothest transition by having the most familiar items in the new residence when your loved one arrives.

Because moving is so stressful, it's not something you want to do repeatedly. Several of my clients relocated their loved ones several times after choosing a community that failed to live up to expectations. If you are planning to move your loved one to a community for the first time, take extra time to ensure a good match. Every new move is incredibly stressful for someone with a memory impairment.

Tip

"Placement agencies" specialize in referring potential residents to facilities, both large and small ("communities"). You do not need to work with such an agency if you choose not to. If you decide to work with a placement agency or an individual specializing in this service, confirm that they will be substantially involved in the process, will meet your loved one, and will work to match their needs with the right living situation.

Many facilities compensate placement professionals for their referrals, so you should expect a high level of service at no cost. Beware of agencies that collect information from you, such as your loved one's name, phone number, and location, in exchange for information. They may provide you with a list of nearby facilities but have likely forwarded your referral information to every facility on that list. You do the work, they get paid, and you lose flexibility in negotiating with any facility.

HOUSEGUESTS

Houseguests disrupt daily routines. Such guests, even when self-sufficient, unintentionally place additional demands on their hosts, which are exhausting for a memory-impaired host. Even joyful occasions like family reunions and holidays are disruptive.

Avoid live-in houseguests wherever possible. Encourage anyone visiting your loved one to stay elsewhere, if possible. Avoid big, lengthy meals. Explain your loved one's memory impairment to guests and offer advice on communicating with them (refer to this book's section on **Holidays**). Look for ways to entertain visitors away from the home and limit visits to 30 minutes or less.

Planning and communicating with intended visitors can save a lot of trouble and avoid adding anxiety or triggering agitation.

HOSPITALIZATION

Hospitalization can cause anxiety or trigger agitation. Anxiety starts the moment an accident occurs, or a hospitalization gets planned. It often grows and becomes less controllable. Agitation may present at any time, including days into a hospitalization when frustration over the lack of familiar surroundings reaches its peak.

Be aware that hospitalization will cause anxiety for your loved one. Mitigate this anxiety using the guidance under **Responding** below.

Tip:

Since hospitalization is effectively a transition for your loved one, and there will be at least one more move at the end of the hospital stay, you may consider moving directly to a new living situation if warranted.

Returning home and moving into a new living situation after-ward is much more difficult for everyone involved.

Changes Related to Caregivers

Non-family caregivers may fill an essential role in caring for your loved one. To you and me, it's their job to care for your loved one. After all, you're paying for their services. Your loved one sees them very differently.

When you hire a caregiver, they become a part of your loved one's life. They may look at the caregiver as a close friend, almost like a family member. While this may be disconcerting, it's natural. The caregiver assists your loved one for days on end. They cook, bring needed items or food, offer feeding assistance, bathe, and help with any number of activities of daily living.

When a caregiver is well-matched to a person needing care, the bond between the two can be constructive and mutually beneficial — akin to a friendship. However, when the match is not optimal, conflict can arise. When placing a new caregiver with your loved one, monitor the relationship between the caregiver and your loved one. Is the caregiver sensitive to the needs of your loved one? Are they attentive? How does your loved one respond to the caregiver?

If the caregiver is not going to work out, make a change as soon as possible to avoid the anxiety that will result from changing a caregiver your loved one has come to rely on for their activities of daily living.

Home Emergencies

Toilets overflow. Sinks get clogged. Electric outages happen without notice. Extreme weather and earthquakes occur. Things break around the home, from air conditioners to washers and dryers to kitchen appliances. Any one of these is annoying to you and me, but to your memory-impaired loved one, it can throw daily routines into a tailspin.

Stay on top of home repairs to the greatest extent possible, and have emergency procedures and supplies on hand to provide as much comfort as possible in the inevitable emergency.

Travel

Think about your last trip, whether by plane, train, or automobile. Was it uneventful? Travel is often fraught with anxiety-inducing situations for even the most seasoned traveler.

Travel is even more anxiety-inducing for your loved one with a memory impairment simply because they are leaving the comfort of familiar surroundings. Even a car ride of 15 minutes to your home can be discomforting. Your home may not be comfortable to them, even if visited dozens of times before. Getting in and out of the car may be a challenge. Negotiating the path from the car to the home may present another challenge. Then, if you have others visiting, there is the stress of forgotten names, and guests dwell on details like the last time they saw your loved one, who does not remember.

If planning an event, think carefully about having your loved one join. Such events are exhausting to someone with a memory impairment. It may be easier to bring Auntie to an event at home, a restaurant, or another location, but it's better to visit her instead. Celebrate holidays early, adapting whatever traditions you enjoy to the new situation. Doing so will help your loved one, but it will also help you enjoy your event or holiday without the guilt of not having them with you.

Threats and Perceived Threats

Recognize that your loved one who has dementia doesn't always perceive things the way you might expect. Often they have been increasingly masking their memory impairment, trying to keep control of their life and retain what independence they can. Even the most innocent comment or action can be perceived as a threat to their autonomy, well-being, or safety, and so cause anxiety or trigger agitation.

Preventing Anxiety

CASE THE SPACE

- Find ways to reduce stress in the environment. Adjust temperatures, find quiet places, play soft music, whatever makes your loved one feel safer or more comfortable.
- Encourage routines, rituals, and habits. People with memory impairment respond well to ritualistic behavior and don't like disruptions.
- Add comfort to the environment. Remember that long-term memory often remains intact even when short-term memory has declined. Family photographs, heirlooms, familiar furnishings, and other objects of personal value help.
- Limit caffeine. Caffeine causes anxiety in memory-impaired adults just as it does in anyone.

AVOID THE TRIGGERS

It may seem obvious, but if you know what triggers agitation in your loved one, avoid those triggers!

In addition to the triggers listed above, other distractions may cause anxiety or agitation. These include noise, glare, and background distractions (such as having the television on even when no one is watching). These may or may not bother you, but they can irritate your loved one. Avoiding these should be top on any caregiver's list.

MONITOR PERSONAL COMFORT

It's easy to overlook the personal needs of those who have dementia. They may not remember the last time they ate, drank water, or had a bowel movement, and often don't complain. On top of that, the generation with the most people with dementia grew up not drinking enough water.

There are a plethora of common symptoms of dementia to monitor and ensure proper care. The Alzheimer's Association suggests checking for the following:

- Hunger
- Thirst
- Constipation
- Full bladder
- Fatigue
- Pain
- Infections
- Skin irritation

When in doubt, consult a medical professional.

Other suggestions from the Alzheimer's Association include making sure the room is at a comfortable temperature, being sensitive to fears, perceived (real or imagined) threats, and frustration with expressing what your loved one wants. Sadly, frustration with the inability to express wants is a common symptom of dementia.

SIMPLIFY EVERYTHING

Seriously, simplify. Forget about new technology and focus on personal interaction. Focus on the essentials. Go for a walk. Garden together. Put on music and dance. Provide an opportunity for exercise. All these can be comforting for your loved one and good for their health.

Responding

Do your best to avoid triggering agitation. However, once anxiety or agitation appears, it needs to be addressed. You need to understand and practice approaches that have been proven successful.

When a person with dementia is agitated, our first instinct is often to try to calm down the person, which rarely works because it doesn't address the root cause. Attempts to calm them may even increase their level of agitation. Although it may seem counter-intuitive, sometimes the best course of action is to back away and give the person some space while still keeping a close eye out to ensure the safety of themselves and those around them.

Many people feel stifled and uncomfortable when there are too many stimulants, including people, around. By providing space, we allow the person to navigate their problems on their terms, calm themselves down, and regulate their own emotions. This sense of control not only helps the immediate outburst, but it can also help them avoid future outbursts and improve their quality of life.

If your loved one is a danger to themselves or anyone else, please seek professional help immediately. Keep emergency numbers handy, and don't hesitate to call for help.

Here are a few approaches to try and master. Not all are relevant for every situation, but all may help your loved one deal with anxiety and agitation.

LISTEN TO THE FRUSTRATION

Don't argue with or correct your loved one. Instead, try to understand what is causing frustration. Use the validation approach and put yourself in your loved one's shoes.

INVOLVE YOUR LOVED ONE IN ACTIVITIES

Offering activities is a form of redirection, taking the focus off the anxiety trigger and directing attention to something else. Music is compelling. See the section on **Confusion and Forgetting** for suggestions on how to use music to tap into long-term memory. Use art or other activities to redirect your loved one away from the anxiety.

Exercise is another way to redirect your loved one and has the added benefit of giving them another outlet for their energy. Go for a walk. If they have difficulty walking, getting them up and into the car for a ride may be sufficient exercise and offer an activity.

VALIDATION AND REASSURANCE

When someone is agitated, don't confront them with questions or arguments. Listen to them and validate their fears, and then offer reassurance. For example, I might begin with, "I'm very sorry you're upset." If I know the cause of the anxiety or agitation, I might offer to stay with them until whatever situation is present is resolved. Reassure your loved one of their safety, that you won't let them suffer harm.

MODIFY THE ENVIRONMENT

Sometimes anxiety is caused by environmental factors. Is there excessive or repetitive noise? Find ways to decrease noise or distractions or relocate to another quieter room.

Often overlooked is television programming. Today's news broadcasts include disturbing stories that someone with dementia can easily misinterpret. If the television is on, watch a happy program your loved one enjoys and avoid television news.

BE ON YOUR BEST BEHAVIOR

From simply asking, "Why?" to directly confronting them with, "Don't feel that way," you may cause anxiety and agitation. Never argue with someone with dementia. Not only will you not win, but you can also do more harm than good in a difficult situation.

Keep calm, and do not raise your voice. Don't show irritation, alarm, or offense at the situation. Other things to watch include cornering, restraining, criticizing, arguing, surprising, startling, or ignoring your loved one.

ICE CREAM

I've used ice cream for years to calm agitation. For whatever reason, ice cream has a near-magical effect on agitation, helping to bring calm so I can use other communication techniques in my tool kit.

SEEK PROFESSIONAL ADVICE

You don't have to deal with agitation alone. Even if you've already seen a doctor to address any treatable medical conditions or underlying pharmaceutical or environmental causes, keep the primary care physician in the loop. If you notice any sudden increase in anxiety or agitation, consult them again.

Also, it's helpful to take advantage of support groups facilitated by someone with experience in Alzheimer's disease or other dementias. If you don't know of any in your area, the Alzheimer's Association (www.alz.org) can steer you in the right direction and sponsors online support groups.

Diana, 78, lived alone in a large home overlooking the Pacific Ocean. She had three sons, only one of whom lived nearby. Phil would visit his mother frequently and find her wandering about her home. He insisted that she calm down, sit, have a bite to eat, and drink some water. Diana mostly refused. She seemed incapable of sitting for more than a few minutes at a time, instead getting back up to wander.

Alone at night, Diana was an accident waiting to happen. Despite living in a single-story home, Diana was still a high fall risk and would be in dire straits without a medical alert system.

Her home was too large for her to occupy alone safely. The open space and boredom contributed to feelings of anxiety, causing Diana to become more agitated. Wandering about the home was the outward sign of that agitation, and the overwhelming size of the otherwise-unoccupied home was daunting.

It took about six months to convince Phil that his mother needed to transition to a community that could better meet her needs. After moving, I made a point of taking Diana on outings about once a week to help her feel more independent and in control of her life. She has been living well in community living now for about two years. Her condition is progressing, and she shows signs of increasing anxiety and confusion. Still, her agitation has decreased, particularly after shifting her room from a busy community wing to one with fewer residents more suited to her situation.

Combativeness

For this chapter, we'll talk about aggressive behavior in general, encompassing the spectrum of anger, aggression, and combativeness as a single topic. In practice, fears and frustration can lead to irritation, aggression, and hostility as the disease progresses, or suddenly when an unknown stressor goes unaddressed.

Understanding

Aggressive behaviors, including combativeness, can occur suddenly and without warning in those with dementia. Often there is no apparent reason for a combative episode, whether physical or verbal. Many things, notably discomfort, might trigger it. If your loved one is in pain, they may act out in a combative manner.

Environmental factors also play a role. Like triggers for agitation and anxiety, combative episodes might be from hunger or thirst, constipation, a full bladder, infections, or any physical irritation. They may also start with a miscommunication between your loved one and caregivers. Yet more triggers are delusions and paranoia that can result in self-defense from a perceived threat.

Anyone experiencing abnormal behaviors should receive medical attention and a thorough medical check-up, especially when they appear suddenly. Treatment of an underlying condition depends on accurate diagnosis and exploring possible causes for the behaviors the person is experiencing.

Combativeness also results from underlying anxiety, so review that section of this book for guidance.

As with all behaviors associated with dementia, the underlying cause is the progressive deterioration of brain cells and memory function. As brain function declines, frustration increases, and your loved one has difficulty tolerating it. At the same time, inhibition diminishes. Without inhibition, frustration can quickly (seemingly unexpectedly) turn into aggression or combativeness.

Preventing

Combativeness can occur routinely or appear infrequently and without warning, often accompanied by underlying anxiety. Recognizing and addressing this underlying condition may help avoid triggers for aggressive behavior.

If the person with Alzheimer's tends to be aggressive, be on the watch for symptoms that might push an underlying agitation into a combative episode. Also, seek medical evaluation to explore possible medical interventions to help prevent future hostility.

Intrusive activities such as assistance with bathing or toileting can also trigger aggressive behavior. These activities are often necessary for health reasons. Still, it's worth exploring ways to help your loved one retain as much dignity as possible, even when assisting with personal daily activities that are conventionally private. Consider same-gender caregivers trained explicitly in these activities. Also, limit the number of different caregivers who help in this manner. When introducing a new caregiver, go slow and build rapport before becoming involved in intrusive activities.

Responding

At the first sign of any behavior change, seek medical advice and a complete medical examination. Medications may temper aggressive episodes, but these do not always work well.

It's essential first to understand what is causing the aggression. Often, combativeness results from frustration over problems communicating needs. When your loved one is in pain and unable to share this, they may become angry and hostile.

Consider these possible causes of aggression:

- Pain
- Infections, notably urinary tract infections (UTIs)
- Not enough sleep
- Hunger or thirst
- Medication interaction or undesirable side effects
- Sundowning
- Overstimulation
- Understimulation (boredom)
- Depression
- Fatigue

UTIs are common in those with memory impairments due to a decline in proper hygiene. UTIs can cause undesirable symptoms, including hallucinations, balance issues, pain, general discomfort, delusions, and more. Any one of these can lead to aggression.

Other response options:

- Focus on your loved one's feelings, not their aggression. What's behind the behavior?
- Stay composed. Speak slowly and calmly and conceal your frustration.

- Be positive. Reassure your loved one that all will be good.
- Keep distractions to a minimum. Let's all focus on a positive outcome without external distractions.
- Use music. See Music under **Confusion and Forgetting**.
- Redirect. Shift your loved one's attention to another activity or conversation topic.
- Take a break from whatever activity is causing the behavior. Toileting, showering, and personal hygiene with assistance can be stressful, so take one at a time.

If all else fails, try something different. Change the time of day for an activity that triggers aggression or change the order of events. Add other elements to the environment, such as music. Maybe it's your approach or something else that your loved one doesn't like.

Combativeness is not a behavior to take lightly. Without malice, your loved one can unintentionally cause physical harm to you, your loved one, or others. If your loved one demonstrates combativeness or shows even minor signs of aggression, seek help from a professional as early as possible to protect you and the well-being of your loved one. Keep emergency numbers handy.

In his early eighties, Paul had been diagnosed with fronto-temporal lobe dementia. He had been increasingly demon-strating symptoms of his disease, including wandering and exhibiting periods of agitation and irritability. His wife, Kitty, dismissed his decline and excused his behaviors as aberra-tions. She instead hid the behaviors from their children even as she stressed over providing his care.

When I first became involved in his care, Kitty told me of finding feces around her property. While initially be-lieving a large animal left this, she quickly realized they were from Paul. Sadly, this was not inconsistent with the socially inappropriate behaviors associated with fronto-temporal lobe dementia.

I recommended that Paul attend a day program at a memory care facility. While at the facility, Paul suddenly crashed his body through the facility doors, and the administrator declared him unsuitable for the program because his condition was not as initially disclosed.

One day, Kitty phoned me at 2:15 in the morning. Paul was combative for no apparent reason, throwing whatever household items he could get his hands on, smashing glassware, and throwing objects through windows. Kitty was unable to calm Paul. I used several techniques described in this book and comforted him. The next day, Kitty transitioned Paul to an assisted living community specializing in dementia care. He lived well in this facility with only minor incidents, handled by the community, until his passing one year later.

Hallucinations

Hallucinations can affect some people with dementia, particularly in the later stages of the disease. They are also symptoms of Lewy body dementia or Parkinson's disease. Although there is a medical aspect to hallucinations, they also lead to behavioral issues that are difficult to address.

Understanding

Hallucinations are experiences where a person senses something that does not exist. These are often visual but may involve other senses: smell, hearing, taste, or touch.

When hallucinations begin to appear, they might be small and quickly dismissed. Your loved one may recognize them as not real. Over time, however, that insight fades, and caregivers are surprised when hallucinations become problematic.

Hallucinations may be a face from the past, a different location, or even voices. They present in many ways and can be pleasant, benign, annoying, agitating, or frightening. In some cases, your loved one may recognize they are hallucinating. In cases of advanced dementia, they can easily mistake hallucinations for reality. In some cases, this can be extremely dangerous for anyone involved.

Hallucinations can result from the changes that dementia causes in the brain. They might also result from mental illness, like schizophrenia, or a medical condition. Other causes could include:

- Diet and poor nutrition
- Dehydration
- Fatigue
- Kidney or urinary tract infections
- Pain
- Vision issues
- Drug or alcohol abuse
- Medication

Responding

MEDICAL ADVICE

When you recognize that your loved one is experiencing hallucinations, seek medical advice immediately. A medical evaluation may pinpoint a cause other than advancing dementia. Bring a complete list of all current medications since they may be part of the problem.

Your physician may recommend medical treatment for behavioral symptoms of dementia, which may or may not include psychotropic medication. Listen carefully to the physician's advice and ask questions. Some of the questions I usually ask about medications include:

- What are its risks?
- What are its benefits?
- Are there side effects? If so, what are they?
- Are there interactions between it and other medications your loved one takes?
- How will it affect her?

The Alzheimer's Association advises that psychotropic medications, particularly antipsychotic medications, are associated with an increased risk of stroke and death in older adults with dementia. Be sure to discuss the pros and cons with the physician.

NON-MEDICAL APPROACHES

Hallucinations can be frightening for your loved one, and they may respond unpredictably, which can be dangerous. Use caution during hallucinations and assess whether the situation is safe or not. Is your loved one upset? Are they agitated as a result? Are they frightened by what they're perceiving? If the situation feels uncomfortable, seek help immediately.

In many cases, however, the hallucinations do not lead to dangerous behaviors. Remain calm, and never argue with someone with dementia. Rather than telling your loved one what they are experiencing is not reality, validate their experience and reassure them. Put your arm around them or hold hands and speak softly, reassuringly. See if you can quickly identify how they are feeling. Are they upset, frightened, or scared? Acknowledge these feelings and let them know that everything will be okay.

Consider whether lighting plays a role if the hallucination is visual and in a particular location. Visual hallucinations are far more likely when the light is low. Change rooms or turn on lights; that may help.

Redirection may also help. Change the topic to something else, such as lunch or an activity. Music is a powerful way to connect with long-term memory and may help redirect the focus from the hallucination to something else.

Sundowning

Sundowning is a term used to describe a set of behaviors—including confusion, disorientation, anxiety, agitation, aggression, pacing, wandering, and yelling in people with dementia—that occurs around sunset or into the evening. Other behaviors may include mood swings, demanding attitudes, suspiciousness, and hallucinations.

Sundowning is a common issue that's related to sleep issues. A person needs rest but can't get it because of uncontrolled emotional responses to the condition. In many cases, we don't know whether dementia leads to poor sleep or it's the other way around. Studies are ongoing to discover whether poor sleep contributes to dementia or whether it's an early symptom.

Understanding

We once thought that sundowning was related to the sun's setting. However, it is not tied to sundown and can occur at any repetitive time of the day. Its causes are not well understood but remain a field of active study. The National Institute of Health suggests that one possibility is that dementia-related brain changes affect a person's "biological clock," leading to confused sleep-wake cycles.

Other possible causes of sundowning include:

- Being overly tired, mentally or physically
- Unmet needs such as hunger or thirst
- Depression
- Pain

- Environmental issues, such as shadows or the room being too hot or too cold
- Boredom

Regardless of the cause, many people with dementia experience sundowning. It can disrupt sleep and the body's sleep-wake cycle, leading to behavioral issues later in the day. It can be a vicious cycle.

Preventing

While not a psychiatric diagnosis, sundowning may have an underlying physiological cause that remains the subject of clinical investigation.

The first preventative response to sundowning is to address each of the possible causes. If it isn't having an effect, try others.

- Reduce stress in the environment. Keep spaces well-lit.
- Keep a schedule. Stick to a routine, especially for meals and bath time.
- Take a regular nap in the early afternoon. A quick rest after lunch may suffice to recharge the brain to function well later in the day.
- Plan activities during the day, especially if this leads to better sleep at night. A passive person is more likely to be restless in the evening.
- If outings are necessary, such as to a doctor's office or your home, do them in the morning.
- Avoid caffeine and alcohol. If your loved one is a smoker, find ways to reduce his nicotine consumption in the evenings.
- Keep dinner light. Move the heaviest meal of the day to lunchtime.
- Reduce activity and stimulation in the evening, including people visiting, music, and television.

A person typically will sundown around the same time every day. Look for possible triggers if they become agitated, anxious, or combative. Environmental factors like annoying noise or other disturbances might affect sleep. Medical conditions such as urinary tract infections or dehydration might also trigger unwanted behavior. If your loved one's behavior is new, visit their primary physician.

Responding

The lines between preventing and responding are blurred in the case of sundowning since most preventions are responses to worsening behavioral episodes late in the day. Without appropriate preventive strategies, sundowning episodes can become unmanageable as the disease progresses.

Even with strategies in place, sundowning likely will continue to creep into your life dealing with dementia. Your loved one may become physically agitated, pacing, yelling, or even becoming aggressive. If this happens, never physically restrain them, which will only increase agitation. If pacing, allow them to pace under supervision. If possible, walk with them to reduce anxiety.

If your loved one behaves in a manner that could be dangerous to themselves or anyone else, please seek professional help immediately. Keep emergency numbers handy, and don't hesitate to call for help.

If your loved one also suffers from sleep issues, be aware that the two may be related. Maintain routines around meals and at waking and sleeping times. Put on soothing music or read when it's time to sleep, which helps establish a peaceful mood before bedtime. During the day, try to avoid caffeine, nicotine, and alcohol. Limit daytime sleep and discourage afternoon napping, which only makes matters worse. Encourage physical activity, such as walks.

Here are a few additional tips to help.

KEEP A JOURNAL

Keep detailed notes about the episodes using the date, day of the week, and time format. What did your loved one do that day? How did they sleep the night before? What were they doing before the sundowning events, and who was around? What happened, and how did you respond? How effective was your response?

Hopefully, you notice a pattern emerges that can help you recognize triggers to avoid in the future.

TRY SOOTHING ACTIVITIES

Music is one of my go-to activities for many situations. Music can mentally transport people to another place and time that is meaningful from the past. Music can redirect their thinking and bring calm.

Other soothing activities might include dancing to music, using aromas or essential oils, introducing pets, doing crafts or art projects, and light massages. Be creative and find what works best for your loved one.

TIMING OF MEDICATIONS

Medicines occasionally cause irritability, agitation, and anxiety or can calm them. Talk with your loved one's physician about the timing of medications and find what works best. Administering medications at certain times of the day may work better than others.

TAKE CARE OF YOURSELF

Be mindful of your stress. You may act or respond differently under pressure than when you are calm. Remember that your loved one may not be able to communicate effectively but can pick up on your nonverbal cues indicating stress or frustration. Pay attention to your sleep and be sure you are getting enough. Often caregivers forego their health to care for their loved ones, which takes a toll. Ultimately, this is not good for you or your loved one.

ICE CREAM THERAPY

I couldn't help adding this option here. I've used ice cream for years to calm agitation. I know it's soothing, and my clients usually respond by calming down.

Luciana Cramer, Educator and Care Specialist for the Alzheimer's Association, suggests ice cream "evokes good memories and brings a sense of nurturing and well-being to the present." She adds, "It can be a powerful tool in soothing a restless brain and promoting good feelings."

I don't know the underlying reasons, but ice cream generally calms an agitated person with dementia.

Suspicions and Delusions

Your loved one may become delusional, holding untrue beliefs that often present as unfounded suspicions. They may accuse you or other family members of stealing from them, even when you take every precaution to prevent it. A spouse may accuse their partner of infidelity even as they stand by them, struggling with the pain family caregivers experience in such situations.

While the allegations hurt, the disease, confusion, and memory loss are the cause. It's easy to take the accusations personally, but the condition is causing the behavior.

Distant relatives, paid caregivers, and people outside the immediate family may complicate your response to the suspicions, especially involving theft of valuables. People with dementia do retain some function and have moments of clarity, so you can't dismiss serious allegations out of hand. Discerning well-founded suspicion from delusion can be difficult.

I deal with delusions and suspicions—founded and unfounded— daily. Money and jewelry occasionally do go "missing." Without a complete inventory and documentation of assets, it can be nearly impossible to separate fact from delusion.

Understanding

Ultimately, delusions and suspicions result from the disease and are very common in its middle to late stages. The delusional beliefs are meaningful to your loved one and confounded by memory loss and confusion. Try not to take it personally. They are struggling to make sense of things as memory and reasoning decline.

Note that hallucinations are not the same as delusions. Hallucinations are the result of sensing things that are not there.

Responding

As always, when new behaviors present themselves, seek medical advice immediately. It is essential to rule out an underlying medical condition. Psychotropic medications may be effective in certain circumstances, but, as the Alzheimer's Association reports, "...they are associated with an increased risk of stroke and death in older adults with dementia and must be used carefully." Discuss the pros and cons of any medicine with the physician before making decisions.

REMAIN CALM

Step into your loved one's reality. Try to understand what's bothering them and be a calming influence.

DON'T ARGUE

You can never win an argument with someone with dementia. Arguing can also backfire, making a delusional person more suspicious of you.

REDIRECT

My favorite response is redirecting someone with dementia to another topic and starting a different conversation. Start a new activity. Play music that brings your loved one to other places and times.

HELP OTHERS UNDERSTAND

Make sure family members and caregivers understand that the disease causes suspicions and false accusations and is not a reflection of them.

REPLACE VALUABLES

I often encounter situations where my client's loved one believes someone stole their valued possessions or money, but the client removed them long ago. Replacing valued items in spirit can help mitigate this situation. Provide costume jewelry or small bills instead.

SIMPLIFY

Another go-to response is to simplify. Don't reason with your loved one using logic or reason. Accept the suspicion and move on.

Three-peat (Repeat)

Your loved one may say the same word repeatedly or ask you the same question you just answered, only to ask it again moments later. Maybe they repeat to the point of annoyance, using the same word in the wrong situation. Replacing words they can't recall with inaccurate ones is a common symptom of dementia and Alzheimer's disease.

In season five of the HBO dramatic series *The Sopranos*, a poignant scene involved a meeting between Tony Soprano and his uncle, "Junior." During this scene, Junior repeats that Tony "never had the makings of a varsity athlete." Tony becomes angered by what he perceives as a deliberate provocation. Later, the police find Junior wandering the streets, looking for his dead brother. The writers created a character displaying two classic symptoms of Alzheimer's disease.

In addition to repeated words or phrases, you may also notice repetitive behaviors in your loved one. They may rock back and forth or fold a paper several times, unfolding it moments later and repeating the fold. When asked why, they deny it, are unaware, or change the subject while continuing the behavior. It's easy to get frustrated, but repetitive motion or speech is a common symptom of dementia.

Understanding / Preventing

There's not much we can do about repetitive speech or behaviors. They may be frustrating but are not usually dangerous or harmful. It is essential to see the behaviors as symptoms of the disease, not as your loved one deliberately annoying you.

Be aware that outside events, encounters, and other situations can trigger or make repetitive behaviors more pronounced. Even though you want to prevent these events, they are largely unpredictable — things happen to all of us. Your loved one may be trying to express fear, concern, anxiety, frustration, or other emotion in response to something out of their control. They may be trying to tell you something important but can't effectively communicate it. Because of this, and the disease's progressive nature, you need to regularly monitor the situation and anticipate your loved one's needs.

Responding

EXPLORE FURTHER

Is your loved one trying to communicate something? Do they exhibit the behavior around certain people or places or at a consistent time of day? If you notice a pattern, explore further.

Ask probing questions. If they cannot answer, try a series of yes/no questions, such as, "Is something wrong?" and "Are you trying to tell me something?". Add more direct questions as you narrow down the possibilities. If you think it may be something in the room, move around and ask if you're close to what they're trying to tell you about. The possibilities are endless in trying to communicate through the disease.

BE PATIENT AND UNDERSTANDING

Don't take it personally or let it bother you. Remember that dementia affects memory; your loved one may not remember telling you something or asking the same question moments ago. Offer reassurance that you understand, or answer again if asked a question. Use a gentle approach — touch and voice.

Never argue with someone with dementia. You can never win.

Answer the Question

If your loved one is repeatedly asking the same question, answer every time in a calm, soft tone. Find ways to relieve frustration. Failing memory doesn't mean your loved one can't read your frustration.

If the answer to a repeated question is important, write it down and post it in a conspicuous place. Place notes in critical locations or use memory aids like photographs or calendars.

Beyond the Words

It's easy to focus on the repetition rather than finding out how your loved one feels. Look beyond the behavior and try to understand what's behind it. Is your loved one nervous or anxious? Are they frustrated? These are common emotions among those with memory impairments, especially as the disease progresses.

Do Something with the Behavior

Sometimes repetitive behaviors involve the hands. If possible, turn the behavior into an activity, like wiping a table. Grab a cloth yourself and do some cleaning together.

Develop a New Hobby

One approach that has multiple benefits is to learn a new hobby. Hobbies are beneficial because they offer a sense of purpose and an avenue for creative productivity. Research suggests that engaging in activities and not watching television all day helps to stimulate the mind. This, in turn, helps lessen some of the symptoms of dementia (including depression and repetitive behaviors) by developing new neural pathways.

Although we think of hobbies as something we choose based on our interests, you can initiate a new hobby with your loved one with dementia. Consider drawing, singing, or learning music appreciation ("name the tune"). Collecting everyday things is a hobby for some, like canceled stamps or envelopes. Scrapbooking need not be a product-focused activity; try cutting items out of magazines and using glue or paste to affix them to construction paper. The list is endless.

Do Something Else

Sometimes your loved one is bored or restless and needs something to do. Play games or read books, keep it light-hearted, and have fun.

Gardening is another activity that offers numerous benefits. It can be done indoors with cups and potting soil, but heading outdoors adds fresh air and sunshine. Gardening is tactile and stimulating, helping reduce many symptoms of dementia, including repetitive behaviors. It can also be rewarding to see and care for plants as they grow under your loved one's care.

Play Music

Music from the past may help or provide comfort.

Accept It and Move On

Especially when the repetitive behavior isn't causing harm, try not to let it bother you and find ways to live with it.

Wandering

Wandering is a behavior exhibited by many with dementia at one time or another. It can be unnerving for caregivers, realizing that your loved one may not be able to find his way "home" if he gets lost or disoriented, even in an area that has long been familiar to him. It doesn't help that television news occasionally highlights stories of someone with a memory impairment who's gone missing, adding to our fears.

Understanding

Wandering may be unnerving for caregivers, but it's not unusual and shouldn't be surprising. If your loved one is ambulatory, they have many reasons for moving about - walking to the refrigerator, going to the store, using the restroom, moving to a shaded place when it's too sunny, and so on. As a result of dementia, your loved one may forget where they are going, can't find familiar things (like the bathroom), or look for something they have no possibility of finding.

Wandering can be benign, but it can also be dangerous. Your loved one can "wander off" and get lost, stumble, or hurt themselves during confusion or disorientation.

Many symptoms of dementia can contribute to wandering, including anxiety, agitation, confusion, forgetting, and hallucinations. Each may trigger your loved one to wander for a variety of reasons.

DISORIENTATION

Your loved one may wake up at night and become disoriented. Did you ever awaken in a hotel room and experience brief disorientation?

That's what it can be like for your loved one. They may be looking for the restroom and essentially get lost. Disorientation isn't limited to waking from sleep. Recognize that your loved one may feel disoriented even in familiar places like home.

CONFUSION

Your loved one may become confused about what seems like simple things, such as the location of the kitchen. They may wander the house looking for something that doesn't exist or someone who isn't there. Confused about where they left their keys, they may be searching for them, even if they don't need them. Confusion can also trigger other symptoms, such as disorientation or agitation, so the reasons for wandering may be challenging to understand at first.

ANXIETY

An anxious person may nervously wander about, pace the hallway, or repeatedly look for something they no longer have. Restless wandering is one way to recognize when your loved one is experiencing anxiety.

AGITATION

Since agitation is often rooted in anxiety, an agitated person may need an outlet for their nervous energy. They may pace, but she may also move frantically about or try to "escape" the confines of her surroundings.

HALLUCINATIONS

People who experience visual hallucinations may wander to escape them. When asked, they may insist on a reason that may make no sense to you. These may be your first warnings of hallucinations.

VISION

Vision is an issue that's often overlooked when dealing with wandering. The mind can sometimes play tricks, and familiar places can seem unfamiliar due to dementia, deteriorating vision, and spacial awareness. Vision is a process involving the brain and is affected by dementia because memory begins to fail.

WARNING SIGNS

Any ambulatory person with cognitive impairment is at risk for wandering. Knowing some warning signs and being on high alert for them is essential. According to the Alzheimer's Association, these include:

- He wants to go home, whether in a new residence or still in his home of 40 years.
- She tries to do things she no longer needs to do, like go to work or the store.
- He is anxious, evidenced by pacing or repetitive motion.
- She is confused about locating familiar places, like the bedroom, bathroom, or kitchen.
- He asks where relatives or friends are (they may even be deceased).
- She takes longer than usual for routine walks or drives.
- He appears "lost" in new places.
- She acts like she is doing a chore or hobby but isn't getting anything done.

Preventing

There are a few things you can do to help prevent wandering. I loosely separate these into *non-physical* measures, which address potential underlying causes, and *physical* measures.

NON-PHYSICAL MEASURES

- **Establish routines**. Routines lead to habitual behaviors. For example, they can help your loved one understand when it's dinner or bath time.
- **Avoid circumstances that can be confusing**. Busy places like the mall or grocery store can confuse and cause disorientation.
- **Address other issues and explore possible triggers and causes**. If your loved one wanders at night, is it because they need to use the bathroom? Limit liquid intake starting a few hours before bedtime. Be sure low-level lighting is available if night wandering is a problem. Many products on the market provide low-level lighting with minimal use of electricity.
- **Hide motor vehicle keys**. Whether or not your loved one is safe to drive, hide the car keys. Always keep your keys safely in your control. If your loved one can't drive safely, eliminate the car keys.

PHYSICAL MEASURES

Securing the physical environment may be an option. If possible, install locks on doors to prevent wandering. Locks should not impede egress in emergencies, however. "Safe" options include:

- **Place locks out of the line of sight** — up high where you don't customarily find such devices. One device requires raising and twisting a simple locking mechanism that easily opens for someone without memory impairment.
- **Disguise doors and knobs.** Painting doors the same color as the walls can effectively camouflage doors. Similarly, paint bathroom doors a unique, high-contrast color to identify them quickly.
- **Use child-proof knobs.** Adults easily open them, but children don't figure them out until later years. The same goes for the memory-impaired.

- **Install alarm devices on exterior doors.** Use alarms on windows if your loved one suffers from hallucinations or extreme agitation. I've run into my share of slippery wanderers who surprise their children with Houdini-like escapes. A simple bell above a door, like in boutique shops, can also work.
- **A bed alarm can alert you or other caregivers to your loved one getting out of bed.** This can be an early warning if your loved one is prone to wandering.

Some communities install button combination locks on exit doors, but this can be dangerous in an emergency. In such cases, everyone caring for your loved one must have the code to exit. **Never leave your memory-impaired loved one locked in and alone.**

Responding

If you find that your loved one has wandered off, remain calm. Once found, suppress your emotions and reassure them that everything is fine. Don't correct them if they want to go home, but you're taking them elsewhere. Redirect the conversation as needed. "We are going home," or "We'll be home soon." "Let's stay here for now. We can go home after we get some rest."

If your loved one wanders often, ask yourself when the wandering occurs. Does the wandering happen at the same time each day? Is it related to the same activity each day? What is the cause, if any? Sometimes lack of engagement — physical or mental — is at fault. Exercise and activity can minimize wandering by reducing anxiety, agitation, and restlessness.

Is there an underlying reason for wandering? Has she gone to the bathroom? Is she thirsty or hungry? I'll repeat here some of the questions with yes/no answers I listed earlier:

- Can I get you something to eat?

- Are you thirsty? Let me get you some water.
- Are you uncomfortable?
- Are you in pain?

You can customize your own set of questions based on your loved one's circumstances.

If your loved one is a risk for wandering outside the home:

- Keep emergency lists: police, hospitals, care facilities, and any friends or others you can call for help.
- Ask neighbors to call if they ever see your loved one alone.
- Keep a recent photo and updated medical information on hand.
- Note dangerous places in your neighborhood. Buildings, tunnels, lakes, sewers, ditches, storm drains, forests, etc. If in an urban environment, where are the closest points of access to public transportation or highways where he can hitch a ride?
- Does she have favorite places to visit? If she wanders away, she may be heading there.
- Is he left or right-handed? Those who wander often follow the direction of their dominant hand.
- Purchase identification jewelry. She may wander without her purse but is less likely to remove jewelry.

If your loved one does wander off, of course, search for them. If you do not locate them quickly (maybe fifteen minutes), call 9-1-1 to report them missing. Inform the operator that they have dementia (or say they have Alzheimer's, which is a trigger word for trained safety personnel). Your loved one is known as a "vulnerable adult." After filing a missing person report, law enforcement personnel will look for them.

The Alzheimer's Association operates a 24-hour nationwide emergency response service for people with dementia who wander or have a medical emergency. The program includes a piece of identification jewelry that your loved one wears.

In a wandering away situation, notify the program after reporting to 9-1-1. Visit www.alz.org for more information and keep any phone numbers handy — in your mobile phone, speed dial on your home phone, and posted in a convenient location such as the refrigerator.

In her early sixties, Leilani had moderate to severe Alzheimer's disease. She lived at home with her husband, Darrell. Their two daughters lived nearby, but each had families of their own.

Leilani would frequently wander, disappearing for hours at a time. Darrell and his daughters would search all the places she used to frequent, often finding her at a local convenience store. Sometimes, however, they would not locate her before she managed to find her way home.

One day, Darrell took Leilani on a journey by plane to a resort community. He took no precautions to prevent Leilani from wandering away. On the last day of the trip, Darrell ran a quick errand and returned to find his wife missing from their hotel room.

After searching, Darrell was out of options. The hotel staff believed that she had taken a taxi to the airport. Panicked, he went straight there and located her. She had purchased a ticket to Boston, thousands of miles from home, cleared security, and was waiting to board.

Caregivers must take wandering seriously to preserve safety while maintaining independence and dignity.

Depression

Your loved one with dementia may suffer from depression. It is common, especially during the early and middle stages of the disease, when they are aware of their declining memory. According to the Alzheimer's Association, depression affects up to 40 percent of people with Alzheimer's. Identifying and addressing depression in your loved one can significantly improve their well-being and quality of life.

Understanding

The symptoms of depression in someone with dementia are the same as those in someone without the disease. However, identifying those symptoms can be difficult because many are also symptoms of dementia.

Consider this list of depression symptoms curated from non-dementia sources.

- Trouble concentrating, remembering details, and making decisions
- Loss of interest in things once pleasurable, such as activities, hobbies, or sex
- Pessimism, hopelessness, and apathy
- Withdrawal from social activities and isolation, which can also contribute to loneliness

Each of these can also be symptomatic of dementia.

I must point out that being lonely can lead to depression and declining health for all ages. People with dementia can be lonely while living among others due to the isolating nature of the disease. For those aging alone, however, studies also suggest that it hastens memory decline.

More than one in four American adults over the age of 60 live alone, according to some estimates. Already suffering from loneliness, their depression can deepen. Their long-term health, and often memory, are at risk.

Other symptoms that are not dementia symptoms, such as feelings of worthlessness, guilt, or persistent sad thoughts, may not be easily articulated by your loved one with dementia. Similarly, many physical symptoms accompany aging, including pains or digestive problems.

Responding

If you suspect your loved one may be suffering from depression, talk with their primary care physician. They may refer you to a specialist, such as a geriatric psychiatrist.

Evaluate and follow all medical advice and administer medications as prescribed, including ongoing monitoring of behaviors and follow-up examinations. Be sure to understand the efficacy of recommended treatment. Explore the benefits versus risks and understand the possible side effects of all medicines. Unfortunately, recent studies suggest only minor improvement in symptoms of depression in older adults with dementia.

Although the medical profession uses a set of criteria to diagnose depression in Alzheimer's disease, there is no definitive test. Professionals base their diagnoses on evaluating symptoms and reviewing medical history, including a review of all medications.

As with any depression, there are non-medical approaches that are worth trying. I recommend the following for my clients when depression is suspected (in addition to professional medical consultation):

- Exercise regularly. Exercise can improve a person's health and sense of well-being.
- Eat a healthy diet. Proper nutrition is always important.
- Maintain a schedule of daily living activities and keep to it. Your loved one will get used to regular bathing, meals, etc.
- Join a support group. My clients attend mine regularly with their loved ones with mild to moderate dementia.
- Plan activities. Activities are essential for the memory-impaired to keep them engaged. See the chapter on **Three-peat (Repeat)** for suggestions.
- Keep your loved one engaged in family activities when possible. Counsel family members to engage with her and use proper communication approaches.

Much of this approach is to help reassure your loved one that he is still valued and respected as a family member, whether he is living at home with a full-time caregiver or in a facility with others.

Hoarding

Hoarding is common in people with dementia or Alzheimer's. Sometimes it's an obvious problem: walk into their living space, and it's abnormally filled with stuff. In many cases, it presents less obviously. Your loved one may hide things in drawers among clothing. While many people have a "junk drawer" in their kitchen, the hoarder has many. They become upset or angry if you attempt to get rid of things.

Hoarding is a problem we must address when it challenges our loved one's safety. Food stashed in bedroom drawers presents numerous issues, from food safety to pest control. Essential items randomly tossed into drawers, boxes, or even wastebaskets may become lost, causing frustration and agitation. In extreme hoarding, the home may be cluttered enough to create trip and fall hazards, attract rodents and pests, and increase fire risk.

Understanding

Hoarding tends to occur in the early and middle stages of the disease, although it may have been a lifelong habit that becomes worse. Hiding may be a simple forgetfulness.

While there are many reasons for hoarding, it may be a response to the stresses our loved one faces with dementia, including the insecurity that comes with the disease, an uncertain future, and losing control over their daily lives. Other causes may include feelings of isolation or boredom that accompany failing memory. Some hoarders may even stash objects to help them remember something or a particular time. Others may irrationally fear that someone is trying to steal from them or that their basic needs will go unmet.

Responding

Considering why a person with dementia accumulates things, some hoarding may provide comfort. We still need to monitor our loved one's hoarding habits, however. We need to do something when it becomes unsafe for them or others.

Here are a few examples of when it's time for us to respond.

- Your loved one stops using their bed or bathroom due to extreme clutter.
- The living space is so cluttered that it's difficult to walk and presents a trip and fall hazard.
- Flammable clutter presents a fire hazard near stoves, appliances, and heat sources.
- Sharp objects like knives, forks, or glass are involved.
- Hidden garbage or food can rot and create health hazards.
- Perishable food may cause disease if eaten.
- Your loved one takes on (or continues to) more pets than they can manage.

If you need to act and reduce the clutter, ask your loved one to help, emphasizing that eliminating it helps them maintain their independence. Unless the situation is extreme, remove only as much as your loved one allows, and don't rush. Consider using bins to help organize the remaining items, and add labels to bins, cabinets, and drawers so your loved one can find things and know where they belong. Another tip is to offer to remove duplicates or similar items saved. For example, ask them to keep one or two can openers or one newspaper at a time.

Many hoarders are uncomfortable parting with their stuff if dumped in the trash. Consider donating them to charity or giving them to a family member. However, remove everything you purge from your loved one's living space. You don't want them bringing it back in!

SAFETY CHECK

While you're helping reduce clutter, it's an excellent time to perform a safety check. Test all smoke and carbon monoxide detectors or install them where needed. Locate and check the charge on all fire extinguishers. If your loved one lives independently in their home, consider a professional inspector to review electrical and other systems, like heaters and appliances.

IMPORTANT ITEMS

Another challenge with hoarding is preserving essential items, like eyeglasses, keys, jewelry, and important papers. You don't want these items to become lost in the clutter. If your loved one has a habit of putting something in a particular spot, endorse it. Add a tray or cup and label it.

Keep a spare set of items used routinely, like eyeglasses, keys, remote controls, and hearing aids. Put them in a safe place your loved one isn't likely to disturb, like a basket on the refrigerator or locked in a cabinet. Locked cabinets mean fewer hiding places, too.

You might need to lock some items in a secure place. Consider using a small safe or locked cabinet for jewelry, cash, and important papers. Leave out only small amounts of money and replace valuable jewelry with costume jewelry in cases of more advanced dementia.

Also, be sure to check wastebaskets before emptying them. As odd as it seems, hoarders sometimes stash items in them, even mixed in with trash.

Keep in mind that people who hoard may resent your efforts and act out irrationally. Monitor your loved one's anxiety level to avoid emotional outbursts or combativeness. If continuing is unsafe, you may need to purge when your loved one isn't around.

If you feel cleaning up a hoarding situation is unsafe, it's time to call in a professional that works with dementia and Alzheimer's patients.

One of my first cases as a care manager required me to evaluate my client's mother, Helen, and her living situation. My client's goal was for me to assess the home and make recommendations for Helen to age-in-place safely.

The house was run-down, and the debris-filled yard was overgrown with weeds. It looked neglected for over a decade. Before I approached the front door, I was concerned about Helen living alone and was afraid of what I would find inside.

Trash filled the living room almost to the ceiling. I couldn't see the floor as I walked through the home, stepping on debris and paper strewn everywhere. Decaying food in dirty dishes covered the kitchen counters, and the air smelled awful.

I saw trash everywhere I looked. Boxes filled with who-knows-what were stacked randomly in every room. Bathrooms were no different, making me wonder how Helen could bathe, toilet, or brush her teeth. A black mold covered the sinks and the bathtub.

Helen's family moved her to a licensed six-bed home where she was well cared for. She continued hoarding behaviors, taking items from the dining table and hiding them in her walker's pocket, nightstand, and drawers. Staff retrieved things weekly without Helen knowing.

Financial Irresponsibility

Not surprisingly, people with dementia begin having trouble managing their finances. On one level, basic math begins to challenge people with dementia due to declining short-term memory. Recent studies point to this irresponsibility starting five or more years before a dementia diagnosis, charting a worsening history of missed credit card and other bill payments, lowered credit scores, and even paying the same bill multiple times.

Severe financial irresponsibility is far more complex, involving other dementia symptoms, including confusion, reduced decision-making ability, loneliness, and boredom. In extreme cases, this irresponsible behavior can wipe out a life's savings and demolish hopes for a comfortable end of life.

Understanding

Unsurprisingly, memory loss and confusion are the roots of challenges with financial management. As short-term memory diminishes, many people with mild dementia develop systems for paying bills. Because the generation most afflicted with the disease in the 2020s is more comfortable with mailed statements, their methods often involve the mail schedule. These systems are also easily disrupted, however. The mail might be misplaced, or bills sent in duplicate. Those with advancing dementia also don't often review the accuracy of charges and seek help only when something is glaringly wrong.

Systems built around electronic payments and automatic checking debits don't seem better and add new wrinkles of forgotten passwords, duplicate billing, and countless email reminders.

For most families and their loved ones, paying bills presents a minor inconvenience. Extreme irresponsibility, however, is far more problematic. While many with dementia continue their past behaviors, including frugality, a few suddenly spend recklessly without regard for consequences. Others fall victim to fraudulent solicitations from evil people and trust too quickly.

I see how gross irresponsibility involves emotion-based symptoms of the disease, like loneliness, confusion, and boredom. The cases I've seen over the years are among the most frustrating I've dealt with. In every case, the person with dementia, even moderate dementia where decision-making is compromised, remained in control of their finances, making legal recourse difficult, if not impossible.

Below are a few specific examples that help convey the seriousness of the problem with financial irresponsibility.

- A pest control company knocked on Anna's door to offer a free termite inspection. She accepted their proposal for several thousand dollars in repairs and remediation. They collected payment and then presented a new proposal to make more repairs totaling over ten thousand dollars. Believing she had no choice but to protect her home, she agreed. I discovered the situation accidentally during a visit, finding the receipts on her kitchen counter. When I investigated, I found no evidence of any work done. Threatening legal action compelled the company to cancel her service order and refund all monies, but it remained in business, possibly continuing its fraudulent activity.

- Don lived alone and admitted to feeling isolated. Large withdrawals and talk of a sudden love interest who lived a thousand miles away in Texas attracted the attention of his adult children, who called me. By then, Don had sent over a hundred thousand dollars to what he believed was a woman in love with him. I alerted the authorities in Texas and directly spoke with a woman who argued that she was in love with my new client despite having never met. I later learned that Don was just one of her victims, and she was likely a tiny part of a larger scheme. The calls stopped, and Don's children took over his finances but never got the money back.

- George borrowed a half-million dollars using his paid-for home as collateral. He began making large charitable donations and boasted how the charities appreciated his support, one placing a plaque in his name. His family was unaware of the size of his loan and contributions until he complained about the monthly loan payment. The bank refused to step in, and rightly so. George was still legally responsible for his finances.

- Keith opened a stock-trading account and began investing in stocks without understanding the market. He bought several automobiles despite not having a valid driver's license.

- Sherry paid her taxes three times. Fortunately, the government returns overpayments.

In every one of these examples, there were warning signs. Families must take steps early to act before it's too late.

Responding

To address common financial management challenges, share financial account details and access with trusted family members. Monitor checking account activity regularly. In worsening dementia, put legally binding systems in place to address the inevitable. Discuss the need for financial oversight with your loved one and get them to sign all documents with a notary while legally able to do so.

I haven't yet addressed the problematic case of family, friends, or caregivers taking advantage of the person with dementia. Because these people are in positions of trust and power over those in their care, only those with legal power of attorney over their loved one's finances can act.

We must help educate our loved ones about the rampant phone, mail, and email scams. Increasing sophistication from the scammers makes it difficult for people with dementia to recognize get-rich-quick schemes or blatant attempts at identity theft. If scammers can fool us sometimes, they can fool people with dementia often.

The most important thing we can do is to spend time with our loved ones and pay close attention. Before any signs of memory impairment, I recommend that everyone take action to protect themselves and their loved ones by establishing financial powers of attorney. I also strongly recommend adding a trusted loved one to bank and other financial accounts. The oversight will make early detection easier.

SECTION THREE

Handling Difficult Situations

THE PRECEDING SECTION of this book dealt with challenging behaviors, which are symptoms of the many forms of dementia. Families often begin coping with behavioral issues before recognizing them as related to dementia long before the diagnosis. People naturally try to rationalize changes in their loved ones based on normal brain function. "She's still dealing with the loss of Dad; this is normal." Or perhaps, "Everyone loses his keys once in a while." Or, another one of my favorites, "Yeah, her memory isn't what it used to be, but it's just a phase. It's normal, right?" So, when our loved one behaves unusually or unexpectedly, it's often a wake-up call for families.

Once their loved one is diagnosed with dementia or Alzheimer's, families find themselves in many new challenging situations. Maybe all family members live out of town and cannot address daily living activities. Perhaps the family wants Mom to live her remaining years at home and is unprepared for all the challenges accompanying that situation. Maybe they are instead dealing with financial issues and struggling to find the most economical way to care for Dad from a dizzying array of choices. Or perhaps the family wants to transition Mom to community living but struggles with guilt or how to tell her that she's moving, even when it's the only logical option to preserve her lifestyle and dignity.

This section of this book deals with various situations that families may face and may need help addressing. I used to assume that families were first required to accept a diagnosis of dementia before addressing most of these situations. I've since learned that people are very willing to go along with learning how to manage difficult situations, even while not accepting that a course of action is required. I've tried to write from that perspective.

While each situation presented here may seem unique and isolated, there are always connections between them when dealing with a dementia diagnosis. Every challenge can guide approaches to others, so read each one while thinking about your situation and that of your loved one.

Living at Home

Almost universally, when families first come to grips that their loved one has dementia or needs care due to challenging behaviors, many new caregivers' first thought is, "How can I keep them safe at home?". That often becomes, "How can I still go to work, and how can I still have a life?". The situation is just unfolding, just beginning, and the disease is progressing. What can you expect to deal with while keeping your loved one safe at home?

Understanding

Families typically see living at home as the "safe" choice. The family home remains the family home. Nothing much has changed, except now the family understands that their loved one needs care and much of it. Their goal is for them to age in place. In dementia, however, families must reevaluate their plan as the disease progresses.

The essential advice I offer families is to stop and consider the nature of dementia. Whatever behaviors your loved one shows, each will likely become more severe as the disease progresses. They may skip meals, or overeat if they forget they've eaten. Wandering will become more risky as long as they remain ambulatory. Gait will deteriorate with age, and they become more of a fall risk. They are at risk for falls or accidents if they forget essential items like eyeglasses or medications. If they seem anxious now, will that turn to agitation or even combativeness in the future?

Living at home with dementia is perilous, especially if your loved one lives alone.

It may be difficult to observe signs of memory impairment. Habitual behaviors in the home can help someone with dementia through typical days but can also mask their impairment. They wake up, shower, and eat breakfast. They go about their daily routine, which has served them well for years, managing their memory loss until bedtime. They may even pay every bill as soon as it arrives in the mail.

Unfortunately, bad things can and will happen when disrupted. Consider the knock at the door by an unscrupulous pest control company offering to treat a nonexistent termite infestation. Think about the so-called handyman who suggests work needed to save the home. I've had to deal with many financially irresponsible decisions to authorize unnecessary repairs that may not even get done. We can't ignore the potential for elder abuse by evil people.

If a spouse provides care, this will tremendously strain their health and well-being. Even the most benign of behaviors become more pronounced over time. Whatever stress is on the spouse now will become more stressful as time passes, affecting their quality of life and, arguably, shortening their lifespan.

Responding

To help your loved one remain in her home (or if you transition her to living with you in your home), you must honestly assess her situation and understand your options.

The risk of a fall at home increases with age, even without dementia. Any fall can substantially reduce the quality of life or even cause death, but those with dementia are even more at risk. Your aging loved one will likely need several physical accommodations to make their home age-in-place friendly. They may need to install grab bars for showering and toileting. They might need ramps or lifts to overcome steps. You must address bathrooms, baths and showers, sinks, non-slip flooring, cabinets, steps, and entry threshold trip hazards. Stairs are hazardous; a fall could lead to severe and life-threatening injury or death. Numerous resources on the Internet offer suggestions for making homes age-in-place friendly. I suggest starting there before turning to contractors who can provide the services you need, if only to guide you on what's possible and practical.

In addition to physical accommodations needed by anyone aging in their own home, your loved one with a memory impairment needs special assistance and care. They will need help with medication management, which is not as easy as it seems. Pill organizers can help, but someone needs to correctly fill the organizers and then make sure that your loved one takes the medicines at the proper time. You can't rely on your loved one to do it for themselves, even if they seem able today.

Below are some care options for your awareness.

- **Periodic caregiving visits** are typically for health maintenance and medication management. This option may be viable for someone in the early stages of dementia with day-to-day care provided by family or others who live in the home or spend much time with their loved one. Call your local hospital and inquire about nurse programs offered at low or no cost, depending on your loved one's medical needs and insurance situation.
- **Adult daycare** may be an option in your area if you are away for extended periods during the day and are concerned about your loved one's safety. Be advised that facilities of this type may not train staff in proper care and how to engage people with cognitive impairments, so do your homework.
- **Daily caregivers** may be an option, especially in mild to moderate dementia. Recognizing that 24-hour care is expensive, many families opt for daily care to keep costs down.

- **24-hour or live-in caregivers** tend to be a very high-cost proposition. Talk over options with local caregiving agencies to determine your best options and explore all viable options. These agencies address all the employment requirements and working schedules. While I can't give financial or legal advice, be aware of tax and employment implications if you hire caregivers directly.
- **Palliative care, hospice care, or comfort care** is essentially end-of-life care. Your loved one must meet specific health criteria to qualify for services, but it doesn't necessarily mean "the end is near." A person with dementia may qualify for benefits nonetheless. Talk with your loved one's physician or care manager for more information.

After considering current and future care needs, families often decide that a transition (move) to a dedicated care facility is in the best interest of all concerned. The cost is typically much lower than 24-hour care and avoids retrofitting homes to become age-in-place friendly. If this becomes the case, refer to the following section on **Moves ("Transitions")**.

Medical Alert System

If your loved one with mild dementia is alone at home, even if you or another caregiver runs to the store for an hour, you should consider implementing a medical alert system. These systems typically use a device worn at all times, such as a necklace, with a button your loved one presses in an emergency. That sends a distress signal to a base unit that connects to a telephone line or cellular service. Depending on the system and your preferences, the base unit contacts you, a call response center, or emergency personnel. Such a system can be a great peace of mind if your loved one lives at home.

Medical alert systems are ineffective if dementia is mild-to-moderate. The person will not know when or how to push the alert button in their time of need. Others may repeatedly test the alert system resulting in multiple 9-1-1 calls. One client was visiting a neighbor and demonstrated how she could press the button to call for help and was then surprised to see emergency services arrive at her home across the street.

Moves ("Transitions")

Moves are a significant disruption but are often unavoidable. They are likely to trigger the behaviors addressed earlier due to the increased stress and anxiety accompanying moving.

Understanding

Many families will one day face the challenge of moving a loved one. When that move is to a residential care facility, we call it a transition. Generally, this option for care is more affordable for people compared with 24-hour in-home care since others share a handful of caregivers. In addition, community living offers social interaction for residents, which is essential for those with dementia.

Moving is disruptive for anyone. It involves a tremendous amount of coordination, frustration, and expense. It also adds anxiety and stress. Planning and carrying out a move for your loved one is no different.

Still, telling your loved one that they are leaving the home they've known for decades and moving to an unknown place can be difficult. They may become agitated or combative and undermine your plans unless you are well-prepared. They may use subtle or blatant manipulation to compound your feelings of guilt.

Planning the actual move may be even more challenging. This section offers advice that may help.

Responding

I advise my clients, "Don't go off the rails. Stay on the ride with me.". If you allow the situation to create unnecessary stress and anxiety (to go off the rails), the transition will not be successful.

A transition has three phases: planning and preparing, transitioning, and becoming accustomed to a new environment. Each has its challenges and approaches.

PLANNING AND PREPARING

Initially, planning a transition is a massive challenge for many caregivers. You're not sure you're making the correct decision, even whether to transition, so it's often tough to start planning. Ultimately you have to answer several important questions for yourself: Is it the right time to transition your loved one? How will I tell them? They haven't been acting like themselves and don't see the danger in staying at home. Will they be angry or become agitated? Will they refuse to go?

Perhaps it's more of *where* to transition your loved one. Am I choosing the right community or home? Will they be comfortable there? Can they (or I) afford it? If so, for how long? These are all valid concerns and cause anxiety while planning a transition.

Are pets involved? Pets often have strong bonds with their owners and vice versa. If your loved one cares for a pet, include it in your planning. Many communities will accept house pets, which can bring a sense of comfort and hominess.

WHERE TO MOVE

Families often tour senior living communities and are "blinded by the chandeliers." They almost always select shiny, new, and well-landscaped facilities over others, independent of the level of care or staff training. Don't get me wrong. Aesthetics *are* essential, and it's vital for your loved one to feel at home in her new environment. Aesthetics will help with the transition and ensure that the decision to move her has her best interest in mind.

The problem with being blinded by the chandeliers is that it's easy to overlook the care your loved one needs and will need in the future. Excellent aesthetics may trump quality of care while your loved one needs minimal assistance with activities of daily living (ADLs). As care needs increase when dementia advances, however, you may soon find the community no longer meets their needs, at least not without tremendous additional cost.

Speaking of cost, explore all costs of moving in and ongoing expenses. Many families fall in love with a community only to be surprised by other community fees or nonrefundable move-in fees.

Instead, seek evidence-based answers related to the level of care. What is the ratio of care associates (care managers or caregivers in some communities) per resident? What training do they have, and how many hours do they receive annually? Are they specifically trained in memory impairment (dementia) or Alzheimer's disease? Are they experienced in handling some of the more challenging behaviors associated with the disease?

You should also explore how and when additional fees apply as care needs increase. Specifically, look at prices for assisting with activities of daily living: incontinence, medication management, showering, two-person assistance getting in or out of bed, and others. Are there transportation fees for scheduled medical appointments? What is the additional cost for someone to accompany him to the office?

Any undesirable behaviors can turn into nasty problems for you during the transition. In many cases, your loved one doesn't understand their need to change care and will do anything—and everything—to protect their perceived independence.

Unfortunately, nothing can prepare you for what I call a challenging move. Sometimes, despite the best intentions and thorough planning, everything falls apart at the time of the move. Mom figures out what's happening and refuses to go with the person sent to accompany her. I've seen cases where transportation arrives, and the driver is wearing a shirt with the facility name and logo embroidered on the chest. Seeing it, Mom develops a stubbornness worse than you've ever experienced. Her determination reaches new heights, and she becomes combative. Police get called, and, ultimately, the transition fails.

MAKING THE TRANSITION

Once you've decided where to transition your loved one, it's time to plan how to make the transition happen. Much of this depends on the disease stage and cognition level.

If your loved one is advanced in dementia, involving them in the transition process may not be good. Presuming you have power of attorney over health and finance, you can make these decisions on their behalf, in their best interests. If awareness of the transition causes anxiety, agitation, or aggression, think twice about using the approaches that require reason. Is telling them in advance that moving is in their best interest, or do you simply want to feel less guilty? If the latter, please review the section on **Caregiver Guilt.** Remember, this should not be about you. It should be about what's best for your loved one with dementia.

If your loved one is in the earlier stages of the disease, many approaches might work, and your loved one will likely be more involved with decision-making. In other cases, it all depends on how dementia has manifested. There is no guide to follow, and much of it relies on instinct or the help of an experienced professional care manager. Your loved one may still have legal rights to choose their living situation. Consult their physician or a neuro-psych (psychologist or psychiatrist) if in doubt about your loved one's mental ability to make reasoned decisions independently.

AFTER THE TRANSITION

Many family caregivers who transition someone to a facility think it's best to continue to visit them frequently after move-in. Often this is the wrong move. It is usually better to allow your loved one time to acclimate to the new facility, develop routines, and meet people. When you visit, you are the one who is "out of place," which leads to confusion and episodes of, "Why did you do this to me?" or "I want to go home.".

Instead, give your loved one time to become familiar with and enjoy their new surroundings. Establish relationships with staff members, and don't be afraid to call to check with them about your loved one's status. Use them as your eyes and ears during the first days to weeks. Ask about their appetite, what they ate for lunch, or whether they enjoyed dinner. Ask about medications to assure yourself all is transitioning well.

When dealing with health concerns, ask for the most senior staff member responsible for residents, such as the Licensed Vocational Nurse (LVN) on duty. If you have issues getting the necessary information, speak immediately with management. You're paying for living arrangements and a level of care. Your loved one is entitled to that care, and you should receive all necessary information to ensure your loved one is receiving that care.

Paying for Daily Care

Whether you help your loved one stay in their home with professional caregivers or move them into a community, you'll likely be shocked at the cost. With inflation, salaries are rising, and caregiving is no exception.

Paying for care is a challenge for most families. Neither Medicare nor private health insurance plans cover assisted living or memory care. Medicare may cover medically necessary care in a skilled nursing or rehabilitation facility for a finite time. Only separate long-term care insurance can make monthly payments for the long-term needs of those with memory impairment, but it must already be in place.

People with low income may qualify for benefits. Exploring this is beyond the scope of this book, but families are encouraged to explore all possible sources of assistance.

Families often need to get creative to find ways to pay for care. It's impossible to cover every possible scenario, but responsible caregivers need resources to work with. With a financial power of attorney, you can evaluate your options based on your loved one's assets that you are likely legally able to use, liquidate, or borrow against. Consult financial advisers and retain legal counsel as needed.

Activities of Daily Living

We regularly shower, brush our teeth, use the bathroom, and probably take daily medications. These are all activities of daily living (ADLs), along with nail care and shaving. We might also include dressing, eating, and mobility on that list, but we'll skip these topics to focus on the most challenging ADLs for adults with dementia.

When children are young, we help them with bathing, brushing their teeth, and changing their diapers. Ironically, our loved ones with dementia often need the same care when the disease leaves them unable to care for themselves. Helping with or performing these activities for our loved ones with dementia, such as a parent or spouse, can be frustrating and embarrassing.

Understanding

As we age, things don't work as well as when we were young. There is some normalcy to this, but nothing prepares us for eventually helping our adult loved one shower or use the toilet. While common, it feels abnormal and uncomfortable, especially when the person needing help is the parent who taught us to be self-sufficient.

Our loved ones with dementia aren't happy about their situation either. They've been self-sufficient for longer than we've been alive and suddenly need help with deeply personal activities. Even in moderate dementia, when our loved one unquestionably needs assistance, they are embarrassed, defiant, and frustrated.

Compounding the emotions our loved ones are experiencing, they may also be frustrated by an inability to communicate their desires and to do as they want. Other behaviors, like aggression, agitation, and depression, can worsen the situation, and the emotions involved can trigger those behaviors. It's a vicious cycle.

Understanding the extremely high levels of emotion surrounding ADLs for your loved one is necessary to respond appropriately. Your frustration will only trigger negative emotions and make the situation worse.

Responding

Of all the situations I address in this book, this one has the most straightforward advice. Preserve your loved one's dignity and self-respect above all else. Put yourself in their shoes and ask how you would feel if you were handled or managed this way. Their modesty is compromised, but you must minimize that to the greatest extent possible.

Below are a few essential considerations when you, or a caregiver under your watch, assist your loved one with their ADLs.

SHOWERING

The discomfort around anyone helping with activities of daily living leaves everyone frustrated, and showering is no exception. Even the mention of bathing or showering can trigger belligerence. Try different words like "freshen up" instead. If your loved one refuses, you may have to step back to allow time and space. Try again later, or use "Creative Dementia Talk." (See **Confusion and Forgetting** for examples.)

Another approach to bathing is to make the activity more positive. Try adding soft music, and don't show your frustration if it surfaces.

Adding casual conversation about the day or other things is a positive distraction from what might otherwise feel like an indignity. Nobody wants to be scrubbed down like in the film, *Silkwood*. Give your loved one a washcloth and ensure they participate in their bath or shower experience, even if you need to guide their hand with yours.

A few specific thoughts:

- Run bath or shower water before bringing your loved one to the bathroom.
- Test the water temperature.
- Even if the bathroom is warm, our loved ones may feel cold. Acknowledge their feelings. Perhaps raise the water temperature a degree or two for the next experience.
- Have all supplies ready before the bath or shower: body wash, shampoo, towels, incontinence care items, and a new set of clothing.
- When rinsing off shampoo, offer a washcloth for your loved one to cover their eyes and face.

ORAL CARE

Sadly, many large and small communities fail when assisting those with oral care. Caregivers struggle with assisting or performing oral care for those with dementia, but it remains essential. Success lies in the approach and understanding of the disease.

Whether caused by age or a disease symptom, people with dementia tend to experience increased sensitivity in their teeth and gums. Soft brushes and toothpaste developed for sensitive teeth can help. Also, avoid using electronic toothbrushes of all types. They feel weird for those new to using them, and the noise can be disturbing and cause anxiety you don't want. Finishing with mouthwash can be refreshing and stimulating if your loved one can swirl and spit.

Dentures are a wrinkle for many adults caring for their parents. Helping remove, clean or soak, and replace them is challenging. Often, it's a question of one problem or another. If you don't remove the dentures to clean them, you risk infection, but your loved one might bite you. Infections are a substantial risk, so talk with a medical professional if anxiety medication is warranted.

TOILETING AND INCONTINENCE CARE

Urinary and bowel incontinence challenge caregivers. On one level, both evoke disgust, which is a natural response. While it may be disgusting, your loved one cannot help themselves, and we need to work past our automatic reactions. If your loved one is incontinent, do not withhold liquids, which can lead to dehydration, urinary tract infections, or other medical issues.

Incontinence can result from not recognizing the need to use the bathroom, forgetting where to find the restroom, infection, or as a side effect of some medications. When incontinence first presents, seek immediate medical evaluation. Possible causes include sleeping pills and some psychotropic drugs, high caffeine intake, or urinary tract infections.

If you suspect your loved one's challenge is finding the bathroom, address the common environmental issues. Make sure bathrooms are easy to locate, even painting its door a bold color. Dress your loved one in easily removed clothing to eliminate fuss when it's time to go. Above all, don't let your disgust show; show empathy instead.

If incontinence challenges your loved one, remember that all responses should consider their dignity. Toileting remains a private and personal situation and will remain embarrassing for them. Don't use terms like adult diaper or even pull-up. "Brief" may be a less offensive term. Significantly, if your loved one does need disposable briefs, change them frequently as necessary, at least five times a day.

Surprising to many caregivers, people in moderate to severe stages of dementia often attempt to play with their feces. Others become constipated and will use their fingers to defecate. If this occurs, I recommend a full-body jumpsuit designed for people with dementia. It prevents them from putting their hands down their pants.

MEDICATION MANAGEMENT

People with dementia struggle to manage their medications like they have difficulty managing finances. Sometimes, people with dementia cling to their medications as a sign of independence. Families often face this challenge in early-onset Alzheimer's or mild or moderate dementia. In my experience, it's more related to when the family recognizes the need for medication management.

Another concern for those with dementia is that they already took a particular medication. Too much medicine leads to bad things. Consider a lock or audible alarm on cabinets with prescription medicines.

We discussed pill organizers earlier. To use them, someone must correctly fill them and ensure your loved one takes the medicines properly, which is the essence of medication management. You can't rely on your loved one to do it for themselves.

Walking, Gait Changes, and Fall Risk

Most of us know that aging also brings challenges to walking if only by the number of walkers and canes we see around retirement communities or care homes. In addition to advancing age, declining physical fitness, strength, endurance, balance, and obesity contribute. Diseases often associated with age can also affect mobility, including diabetes and arthritis. Some estimates suggest more than 20 percent of adults over eighty use at least one mobility aid.

Dementia adds complexity to the mix. Changes in the brain can cause challenges with balance, visual perception, and other senses that affect walking. Indeed, ongoing studies suggest that changes in gait – how a person walks – may be early warning signs of cognitive decline and the onset of dementia.

Understanding

Shopping and other errands are part of our daily lives, so mobility is essential for independence, especially as we age. Even the activities of daily living we discussed earlier in this book require mobility, if not walking. Preserving mobility by minimizing fall risks becomes increasingly important to an aging person's independence and function.

Age is a significant risk factor for a collision with furniture or a catastrophic fall that leads to a bone fracture. Those with dementia are at increased risk due to confusion and forgetting, and many other behaviors and situations associated with the disease. In addition:

- Vision issues contribute to risk. If your loved one has difficulty judging the depth of steps or seeing uneven landscapes or changes in floor texture, the risk of falling increases.
- Judgment also can decline with age. I've worked on countless cases where someone made a poor choice, almost to spite their condition. They insist on climbing steps or walking without assistance, with disastrous results.
- Other risk factors include medications. Discuss living conditions, excessive clutter, or the presence of steps with your healthcare professional.
- Gait and balance changes contribute significantly to increased fall risk.

Gait is essentially how a person walks, and virtually all persons with dementia exhibit changes. They begin walking more slowly, taking shorter strides as they struggle to focus and concentrate while moving. Even seniors without dementia may fear falling, but those with dementia often experience slower stride each year and declining memory function. The brain is the control center for our bodies, and when it falters, it struggles to give adequate signals as before dementia.

By the late stages of dementia, patients lose most, if not all, mobility.

The causes of slowing gait are varied but include visuospatial decline, poor judgment, environmental clutter, medication side effects, fatigue, and pain. Discomfort from needing to use the bathroom, hunger, thirst, and restlessness can all affect walking and balance.

Responding

We should all monitor changes to our loved one's gait, even if we are unsure whether they show mild cognitive impairment. They may shuffle when walking or lean to one side or forward. They may take longer to walk from room to room or stumble over obstacles they could easily avoid. Some begin furniture walking, using furniture around the room for balance as they move from chair to table to sofa.

Family caregivers who live with their loved ones may not notice small changes over time. Modern technology can help. Record your loved one walking occasionally and review the videos once a year. Visitors may also note changes you don't, simply because they aren't familiar with the gradual decline you could easily miss.

One simple test is the "get-up-and-go test" for gait and balance if your loved one complies. The decades-old test amounts to standing up from a chair, walking ten feet forward and back, and sitting again, all without using arms for support. Successful performance in less than ten seconds is the standard benchmark for success.

If your loved one shows changes in cognitive function, movement, and walking, discuss them with your loved one's doctor as soon as possible. These may be early warning signs of dementia you should not ignore.

People with dementia are at greater risk of falls, a real fear and a genuine threat to future mobility. Our loved one might fracture a leg or hip, suffer a head injury, or worse. We can help by ensuring rooms and pathways are well-lit and obstacles-free. We might add visual cues to interior paths, like aligning sofas and chairs to point the way.

As gait deteriorates, ensure safe footwear, such as non-skid shoes with hook-and-loop fasteners. Consider injury-saving clothing with built-in padding in hips, thighs, or tailbone.

Dementia is far more complex than memory loss. Your patience and attention are essential.

Driving

We fondly remember at least one car in our life. An automobile means freedom and autonomy. Learning to drive is a rite of passage for most. Driving became synonymous with independence when the automobile appeared more than a hundred years ago.

Motor vehicle agencies and insurance companies recognize that aging brings slower reflexes and compromises decision-making skills. Dementia further compromises both reflexes and decision-making, complicated by risks of confusion. The news reports of people hurt or killed by confused elderly drivers warn us not to allow our loved ones with dementia to drive. However, when adult children, concerned caregivers, or even government authorities threaten to remove the keys, the person with dementia sees it as a dagger to the heart of their independence.

Understanding

Driving sometimes takes on added significance to a person with dementia. As other faculties fail, they cling to those things they know well, and since driving is mainly habitual, it is often an activity that seems unaffected. Driving also provides a sense of independence, self-reliance, and freedom at a time when the disease threatens those same feelings. Losing the privilege to drive is disturbing and a burden on the family that now must take loved ones to appointments, visit friends, or other places. It may also limit a family's independence, being unable to travel alone.

As the disease progresses, independence becomes more and more attractive, and it may seem there is no apparent decline in driving ability. Make no mistake: driving requires quick decision-making and action. Independent of progressive dementia, age alone slows reaction time. Safe driving requires good motor skills *and* cognitive skills. The person with dementia *will* eventually become unable to drive. You don't want to learn this after a severe incident.

Some people with dementia recognize the risk of driving and stop independently. In my experience, this awareness comes after one or more fender benders or close calls.

Others don't recognize the decline in their driving ability. They don't think beyond routine trips and insist on driving despite the risk. Many of the behaviors of dementia may trigger unexpectedly while behind the wheel. An emergency vehicle, a reckless driver, an automobile malfunction, or any other possible incidents could lead to confusion and anxiety.

Responding

Anyone with dementia should not drive due to the inherent risks. Managing an automobile may be habitual, but people with dementia can quickly become confused, stressed, and disoriented, even driving short distances along familiar routes. Keep in mind every driver shares the road with others. Nobody can predict what might happen on any given trip.

Still, clients ask when they should take away the keys. If they need to ask, the answer is probably now. Indeed, a formal diagnosis of dementia should immediately end driving privileges. Continuing to operate a vehicle is grossly negligent and puts everything at risk.

For the undiagnosed, the answer is more nuanced.

I don't suggest getting into a motor vehicle with your loved one showing signs of dementia at the wheel. Many do, however. Here are a few signs that it might be time for your loved one to stop driving.

- When you notice fresh damage to your loved one's vehicle
- If you see significant changes in their driving habits
- When driving becomes exhausting for them
- If your loved one or someone else reports one or more near-accidents
- Other people are uncomfortable riding in their car
- They are uncomfortable driving at night
- They have difficulty seeing

These are warning signs we must take seriously. If you spot damage to their vehicle, look around the garage and surrounding area because it may have happened nearby. Ask about the dent or scrape. If they won't or can't answer, it's probably time.

Usually, people who note changes in driving habits or become uncomfortable being a passenger in their loved one's vehicle know when driving should stop. For many, a key deciding factor is whether they would allow their children in the car. Pay attention to the vehicle's position in the lane. Note slow responses, poor decision-making, going too slow or fast, and becoming distracted or confused.

If you hear reports from others, take them seriously. Ask for details like the ones you would evaluate yourself if you were in the car.

If you know others have been in your loved one's car and you trust their opinion, ask them how it went. This conversation should be casual and not alarming. You're asking for an assessment for your awareness, not sounding the alarm or implying that driving with your loved one was unsafe. If you feel it is, take away the keys.

Continuing to Drive

Unfortunately, many who know their loved one should not continue driving don't immediately prevent it. Some try but fail. Others are afraid even to try.

At a minimum, have the conversation about driving, even if your loved one will continue. Speak eye-to-eye to emphasize its serious nature. If your loved one becomes agitated, take a break and try again another time.

You may persuade your loved one to go to the motor vehicles department with you for a refresher course for senior drivers. Some insurance companies offer discounted rates for those who complete such courses. Regardless, when your loved one says they are confident in their driving, they should be able to prove it.

Even if your loved one continues driving, explore and try alternatives for transportation. Look into senior transportation services available at low or no cost. Ride-share services may be an option depending on your loved one's ability to use modern phone apps, and you may be able to share their account to monitor use. Every avoided trip behind the wheel helps, and experience using alternative transportation makes them attractive alternatives when driving stops.

Taking Away the Keys

Most experts agree that the time to start talking about taking away the keys is long before it's time to take them away. If possible, have this conversation with your loved one early when the threat of losing a car is on the horizon. The early discussions make later conversations easier.

Many people caring for loved ones with dementia haven't had conversations in advance. They may find allowing their loved one behind the wheel easier than taking away driving privileges. After all, they don't want to upset Mom or Dad, not to mention they would then have the added burden of arranging for transportation.

In cases of early dementia, reasoning may work. Driving is a shared responsibility with everyone else on the streets. They may accept the risk of driving themselves but not think about others on the road, many with poor driving habits. If your loved one has grandchildren, ask if they would be comfortable driving with them as passengers.

Without a diagnosis of Alzheimer's or other dementia, you may be unable to deny your loved one the privilege of driving without their permission. With a diagnosis, their physician can help. Many notify motor vehicles departments, which respond by suspending driving privileges.

CREATIVE MEASURES

If your loved one has moderate to severe dementia, they should never drive. Having missed the opportunity to remove the vehicle with permission during earlier stages of the disease, you may encounter tremendous resistance. If so, you might use a creative approach. Many of these would be considered underhanded were it not for the seriousness of keeping an unsafe driver off the road.

Without legal authority, you should never seize, damage, or modify anyone's property, including a vehicle. If necessary, contact your motor vehicles department. They should have a process for referring a driver for evaluation. You must identify yourself and your relationship to the person you're reporting. You might request confidentiality, but you cannot make the report anonymously for apparent reasons.

With that disclaimer, I've seen a few successful creative approaches.

- John fabricated an excuse to borrow his father's car. He returned without the vehicle. John then redirected the conversation each time his dad asked about it. Over time, the questions stopped.
- Erin took her mom's vehicle for routine service. When Mom asked about the car, Erin reported that it required additional repairs and that parts were on order. Mom eventually stopped asking about the vehicle.
- Abby disconnected the battery in her dad's car. When he tried to use it, it failed to start, and he returned to the house. Abby had the vehicle towed and used Erin's fib above.

These somewhat underhanded approaches worked because of the nature of moderate to severe dementia. Out of sight is out of mind when short-term memory diminishes. If you remove a vehicle that your loved one has been using routinely, a new routine of not using the car will emerge over time. During this phase (and as a general rule), never leave the keys to any vehicle lying around for your loved one to find. That may lead to a new and scary situation.

Allison, 85, had lived independently since her husband passed away fifteen years earlier. Every day at 4:00 PM, she would open her garage for neighbors to gather for an hour of conversation and wine, after which she returned to her solo routines.

Allison still drove her 1985 sedan to familiar places in the neighborhood—the grocery store, the gas station, or the department store. She even passed a safe-driver test with the motor vehicles department.

Allison's routines served her well until the disruption.

While making a routine trip to a store, Allison's car overheated, with steam billowing from under the hood. Confused, she continued driving and became disoriented, ending up at a service station ten miles off course.

A kind stranger drove Allison home. Allison could not recite her address but was able to point the way. She opened her garage promptly at 4:00 PM and returned to her routine.

The family learned of the events days later when Allison wanted to use her car. The family located the vehicle thanks to an address the kind stranger had written down and placed in Allison's pocket. The car's windows were down, the doors unlocked, and Allison's purse remained on the front seat.

Allison and her family were fortunate that nobody was hurt. The vehicle was a complete loss, allowing the family to finally and permanently take the keys.

Caregiver Guilt

Guilt is a common issue that many families face. It can come from any number of situations, including feeling guilty for:

- Making decisions for Mom or Dad or spouse
- Moving their loved one to a community
- Not visiting their loved ones enough
- Confronting a loved one's anger or resentment over a decision
- Failing to recognize advancing dementia sooner
- Disrupting comforting routines and familiar surroundings
- Taking control of finances, involving medical and legal professionals
- Selling the house and belongings after moving a loved one to a community
- Making end-of-life decisions and advance directives on medical forms
- Not spending time with their own family
- Enjoying holidays or times away from their loved one

Caregiver guilt may not be avoidable, but we can better understand and overcome it.

Understanding

Much of the guilt family caregivers experience is rooted in a role reversal. Parents understand that they will make decisions for their children, who grow up and become responsible, independent adults. Most adults are unprepared when they flip roles and assume responsibility for a parent or relative. Additionally, many choices are complex and irreversible. They are also often made without involving our loved ones, which can also feel underhanded, adding to guilty feelings.

Guilt can be overwhelming, affect the caregiver's health, and even lead to psychiatric issues.

Responding

First, we must remember we are making the decisions for our loved ones because they can no longer decide for themselves. Everything we do is in the best interests of our loved ones. However, this is seldom enough to get over unnecessary guilt.

Let's look at some guilt-mitigating strategies.

- **Check your expectations.** Family caregivers often believe they can take on the added responsibilities while continuing their other adult responsibilities. Others want a particular outcome for their parent that is not within their financial resources. Most children who become responsible for a parent want them to be happy with every decision. All of these are unrealistic expectations and not worthy of your guilt.
- **Reflect on your successes**. Many caregivers fail to credit themselves for solving a problem and instead focus on their loved one's complaint about the chosen outcome. A transition from home to a care facility often solves several issues, but then Mom complains and adds guilt over transient situations like becoming familiar with the new living arrangements.
- **Join a support group.** Although no two situations are alike, there are many similarities. People join support groups to share their pain and get advice but also learn from others they are not unique in their feelings. Sharing your guilt with others

caring for their loved ones is often met with a chorus of reasons you're being too hard on yourself.

- **Be proactive.** Addressing situations before they turn critical allows more time to assess options. You're much more likely to be confident in a decision if you have carefully considered options than if you are reacting to an emergency needing immediate resolution.
- **Make time for yourself.** Caregivers overwhelmed by their responsibility can lose themselves in their situation, which isn't healthy for them or their loved ones. They also frequently feel since they care the most, they are the best person to provide care instead of letting professionals do their jobs. Self-care is vital. Take several breaks during the day for yourself, and lower your expectations. You can't live up to them. Keeping a journal can help, and it chronicles a history leading up to and out of critical decisions you can look back on.
- **Complete a Physician's Orders for Life-Sustaining Treatment (POLST).** This document, intended for patients with advanced illnesses like moderate to severe dementia, details care and limits on treatments performed. It is always created collaboratively between a physician, the patient, the person holding power of attorney over the patient's health, and sometimes the patient's family. It can avoid extensive treatments if unwanted and help mitigate guilt by representing a shared decision.

Don't allow guilty feelings to creep in when you have reached your limits. Securing in-home care or moving to a care home or facility is often a better solution for your loved one and lets you return to caring for your physical, mental, and emotional health.

Dump your guilty feelings as best you can. I use a dump truck filled with guilt as a metaphor. Let that truck dump its load and free up your emotions. If necessary, see a licensed psychologist who can help.

Holidays and Extended Visits

End-of-year holidays are when families across the United States or worldwide gather, often seeing one another for the first time in years. They're also a time of stress for families, including financial pressures associated with travel, compounded by inevitable family drama.

Holidays generally bring additional stress for families caring for a loved one with dementia. The financial, time, and task stresses of caring for a loved one intertwine with the nostalgic feelings of holidays past, challenging presents, and fearful futures. Family gatherings further complicate the emotions when many family members see firsthand the effects of dementia on their loved ones.

Extended visits, at any time, seem like they should bring welcome relief for caregivers. Extra hands can help with care or attend to household chores while you're busy caregiving. Unfortunately, most visitors aren't prepared to assist. Instead, they dwell on the negative aspects of the situation in conversation. If they do offer to help with other chores, they interrupt with questions constantly. Instead of relief, most caregivers report stress from the added responsibility of managing their guests' experiences.

Understanding

Most of us have strong emotions associated with holidays. Many people are nostalgic about good memories, but some associate the time with sadness due to life events that don't care about the calendar. Reports of depression tend to rise during holidays. Depending on the nature of your loved one's dementia, they may also experience good or bad feelings around the holidays.

We must understand that we're operating in a new reality and must avoid false expectations based on the past. Doing things the way we once did, including holiday traditions and family gatherings, may not be practical, feasible, or necessary. We can probably simplify many of our customs and still find joy in them.

We addressed guilt earlier, so let's agree we should not feel guilty for declining invitations or simplifying traditions, including family gatherings. We are not alone in wanting to recapture those warm memories, but our realities don't align with those expectations.

Another consideration is how much you tell your guests about your loved one's dementia and declining health. If you tell them nothing, they may feel caught off guard or break down emotionally in front of your loved one. Informing or coaching guests in advance can help, but your guests are likely unprepared for a loved one not remembering details from the past, repeating things, or showing any of the behaviors we've already discussed. Remember your struggle learning to cope with the disease and understand they do what you've learned to do without coaching.

Responding

Since we cannot change the reality of our situation, we must adjust our expectations. We can help our visitors understand and adapt theirs when we've adjusted our own.

As we dementia caregivers know, routines help to maintain balance in daily life. Altering patterns can result in agitation, combativeness, or loss of appetite and illness. Gatherings, house guests, and even holiday celebrations are disruptions. Think through the plans, adjust to minimize their impact, and don't bend to pressures from people who don't appreciate your challenges.

If disturbances are inevitable, keep groups small and downsize plans. Larger groups may cause anxiety in your loved one as noise levels increase, and some faces may not be recognizable. Ensure all guests understand basic facts about your loved one's memory. Explain the situation as well as you can so guests are not surprised when their loved one asks who they are or calls them the wrong name. Offer advice privately, like coaching not to ask if their loved one remembers an event or the names of people in photos from the past.

Addressing extended house guests, never let them make plans without clearly explaining the situation they're walking into. Tell them your expectations if you expect their help, and don't be afraid to say how much work it is. If you don't need their help, or they can't, be sure they understand you expect their patience as you attend to your obligations.

HOLIDAYS

Even in mild dementia, the joys once felt around holidays are no longer the same. Like any of us, your loved one may feel a sense of loss, anxiety, or holiday blues. The joys may be smaller, shorter, yet possibly have more profound meaning, if only for a moment. Patients with dementia operate in "today mode." We are not depriving them of joy by not recreating a past they don't remember well. Enjoy the small moments.

If you plan a gathering of any size, consider incorporating activities appropriate for your loved one to join. Uncle James may be happy drinking beer while watching the holiday bowl game, but that's not a stimulating activity for a person with dementia. Some appropriate activities include:

- Decorating homemade greeting cards
- Looking through family photos or heirlooms while describing each (without using the word "remember")

- Decorating homemade or store-bought sugar cookies
- Crafts, like stringing pieces of loop-shaped cereal or making paper garland
- Wrapping gifts together
- Helping in the kitchen if safe to do so, like rolling cookie dough or pie crust
- Listening to holiday music

If your loved one with dementia lives in a community, think twice before removing them to join your gathering. That trip can lead to many unwanted behaviors. Communities typically host a few low-key events around holidays for residents and often invite family members. Join those instead. They will be nothing like an event you plan based on your traditions, but most residents are happy around others who are happy and enjoy them nonetheless.

If any guests want to visit your loved one in a residential facility, encourage it. If you have concerns, go with them. Check with the home, especially around holidays, to avoid being surprised by walking into a planned activity. Likewise, follow their guidelines for guests. Large groups might separate into smaller groups and visit in a rotation to avoid overstimulation and confusion.

As most people helping a loved one through dementia know, the only time is the present. Celebrate holidays for what they are, but in the here and now. Focus on enjoyment for everyone, including your loved one. The greatest joy may be simply to be with those we love.

Sex

Sex and sexual intimacy are significant parts of our lives. Our loved ones with dementia are no exception, despite changes in their brain, unwanted behaviors, and reduced sexual function. The complexities of Alzheimer's and dementia cause many observable changes, but habits, routines, and long-term memory persist. Factor in hormones and instinct, and you quickly see why dementia, or its diagnosis, doesn't mean the end of sexual activity.

The topic may be uncomfortable, especially when our loved one is a parent. Nonetheless, we must understand it as we prepare for the unexpected, even if we don't openly discuss it with Mom or Dad.

Understanding

People with dementia undergo behavioral and emotional changes due to the disease that affect their feelings about intimacy and sex. Despite this, many couples remain sexually active long after one partner is diagnosed with the disease. Many factors can affect what they consider as sex, however, with some couples spending more time being physically intimate without intercourse.

Other couples may have a difficult time, most often when the healthy spouse is male, and the person with dementia is female. The responsible caregiver loves his spouse and obsesses over providing the best care for her, but what happens if the couple becomes intimate and his spouse becomes agitated or confused? While she may be unable to make some decisions, she retains her right to withdraw her sexual consent, just as she keeps some rights to give that consent.

A central issue is the conflict between a person's right to sexual expression and the disease affecting reasoning and behavior. As caregivers, we must monitor nonconsensual behavior and ensure that our loved ones—and their possible partners—are not exploited.

While physiological differences between men and women lead to some generalizations, either gender may experience changes in their sexual desires as the disease progresses, including a decrease or increase in libido. Some become less interested in sex. Others may become more interested or engage in sexual behavior with others who are not their usual partners.

Sex and the Person with Dementia

While people with dementia have rights to sexual expression, the question is, at what point do they lose the ability to consent to have sex with someone else? Laws might dictate an age of consent for young people, often sixteen or eighteen years of age, based on other factors, but they don't dictate the point at which someone loses the ability to give sexual consent based on the stages of dementia.

Using extremes may help with our understanding.

- A person unaffected by the disease pursuing someone diagnosed with dementia is not okay. This reeks of someone taking advantage and exploiting the person.
- A person with dementia pursuing someone unaffected by the disease is often not okay. Who's to say who is the pursuer in this case?
- Two people with dementia who become intimate, likely in a facility where they reside, is not okay in most circumstances and should be addressed as rape. They moved to a facility for a reason, and while they have rights to sexual expression when it doesn't infringe on the rights of others, they probably don't have the right to consent to sex. Legal remedies

are unlikely, however, which puts the burden on facilities to monitor this behavior.

Where things get muddier is with those who live independently or with family before diagnosis, often in the milder stages of the disease. Without a formal diagnosis, your loved one probably has the legal right to consent to sex, even if you feel they no longer have the moral right. If you find this unacceptable, talk with your loved one's doctor and get them evaluated. If you fail, you have no legal recourse.

INAPPROPRIATE SEXUAL BEHAVIORS

So far, we've addressed sexual intimacy and sex between two people. Some people with dementia develop extreme, inappropriate behaviors that challenge caregivers. Some make sexual advances toward others, almost indiscriminately. Others confuse a person with their partner, leading to a chaotic situation. Some even confuse activities like bathing and personal care for sexual advances. Welcome and unwelcome attitudes lead to wildly different results!

More extreme behaviors include:

- Making vulgar comments or talking freely about having sex
- Taking off their clothes and walking around naked
- Touching themselves in private areas or masturbating in public
- Attempting to touch others in private areas

Responding

Responses to sexual activity between adults with the legal right to consent, meaning pre-diagnosis, are limited. Get a diagnosis if you want to stop it. If you have that diagnosis and your loved one lives with you, you might be able to intervene legally. Consider transitioning them to a community if the behavior doesn't stop. Also, see the chapter on financial irresponsibility and make sure your loved one isn't a victim of financial abuse.

If you observe your loved one making inappropriate sexual advances toward others, consistently remind them it's not okay. Perhaps they only express a need for physical touch, which is increasingly vital for people as they advance in the disease.

If your loved one lives in a community, talk with management about their policies on sex and intimacy. Memory care facilities, in particular, should have strong guardrails to prevent this since all their residents are likely unable to give sexual consent. They may allow appropriate touching, like hugging and hand-holding, which may comfort them.

Remain calm if your loved one acts out inappropriately in public. Some behaviors are not purely sexual but stem from discomfort or a need to use the toilet. Others might be long-standing behaviors done privately for decades, like walking naked around the house.

Distract them by giving them something to do. Offer them ice cream and drape them with a robe. If that doesn't work, see if you can get them into their room or a bathroom. However, if they become combative, take appropriate steps, as discussed earlier.

Sandra is a female resident with moderate dementia. She frequently removes her clothing and walks around her community naked.

While shocking and inappropriate, that was the extent of Sandra's unwanted behavior. Staff members learned to redirect her with compliments about her beauty and guide her to her room, where they could dress her.

Some days this repeats several times but has not led to significant issues.

Caring from a Distance

Caring from a distance is one of the more common challenges I encounter in my practice. It's not that it's the most common situation for families dealing with a loved one with dementia. Still, it is one situation where families quickly realize they need the help of a professional to act as their eyes and ears in town when they can't otherwise be there. As a care manager, I stand in for families in many situations involving their loved ones when they can't be there themselves. I also help translate what medical professionals say and recommend health options or activities of daily living in the context of complex family dynamics.

Moving away from Mom and Dad is more common than ever in today's global economy and increasingly connected society. Children grow up and start their careers, moving out of town, out of state, or even out of the country. Often, adult children are unaware of their parent's diminishing mental capacity and other symptoms until reuniting for some time. Nothing amplifies the symptoms of dementia more than an extended period of absence when the signs stand out like lightning, illuminating the darkness on a stormy night. When the children finally learn what's happening, they can't easily uproot their lives, jobs, or even the businesses they've created. The distance presents unique challenges for caring for loved ones with dementia.

Often, the first outward signs of diminished mental capacity are brought to the attention of families by a medical emergency of one type or another. From a location beyond a conveniently traveled distance, family members cannot offer more care for their loved ones.

Understanding

There are two significant issues at play here. The first relates to being unprepared to deal with your loved one's condition, which is common in today's dispersed family dynamics. It may be a phone call from a physician or concerned friend who reports Mom's memory decline or unexplained behaviors. It could be the first visit in a year, and the symptoms are far more pronounced relative to the last visit.

Many family members feel guilty for not being there to see the progression of the disease, but this brings us to the second issue of becoming aware that your loved one has dementia, regardless of how close you are to them. This issue might be the elephant in the room because recognizing the effects of memory impairment and its related symptoms can be difficult whether you live next door or half a world away. Whether interacting by telephone or in person, Mom can mask her impairment. She may want to protect you, but, more commonly, she intends to preserve her independence. Regardless, living nearby doesn't necessarily make recognizing symptoms of dementia any easier than living thousands of miles away.

Once you know your loved one has a memory impairment, you must understand that the condition will only worsen over time and never improve. You need "eyes on the ground" to check in frequently with your loved one and report back to you—with honest updates. Moreover, you must verify that paid caregivers provide the care you expect and likely pay for.

Responding

The single most important recommendation for families, when no one can routinely check on your loved one and assist with activities of daily living, is to find local help. That help could be a family friend, extended family member, or a paid professional. Caregivers must manage medications, ensure they are in ample supply, and see that your loved one takes them on time and in the correct dose. Depending on the level of involvement, care may also include helping with activities of daily living, such as eating, dressing, bathing, hygiene, and toileting.

If care needs are significant, you may have two choices: living at home with assistance or transitioning to a different situation. Review those chapters if they apply to you.

When caring from a distance, it is essential to recognize that the disease will progress even with the best care from medical professionals and will not get better, except for some relief from symptoms with certain medications. Whatever care needs are now, they will almost certainly become more demanding with time. If using a family friend or other relative, be aware this person or these people are committed to you and your loved one for the duration of their condition. When in doubt of their abilities, contact a professional and have a backup plan in place.

If you need the services of a professional care manager, be sure to do your homework. Ask around and ask for references—and call them. Recognize that some people leave "average" reviews when afraid of repercussions, especially if their loved one continues in their care. Look for glowing testimonials with comments like "would recommend to others."

You must also think about how to pay for care in the long term. While Medicare or other insurance may pay the costs of medical treatment for Alzheimer's or other dementias, they don't usually cover long-term custodial care. Only a preexisting long-term care policy pays for this care.

If caring from a distance, consider the services of a professional fiduciary, especially when multiple siblings are involved. It's good to have someone not directly involved with one or more family members. The fiduciary can work with the care manager in various situations, from broad oversight and reporting to serving as power of attorney for finance or health.

Palliative Care, Comfort Care, and Hospice

Many people think of or use the three terms in the title of this chapter interchangeably. They're all care provided near the end of a person's life, and many people responsible for their loved ones panic at their mention. However, they are not the same, nor do they specifically mean "the end is near."

Understanding

Palliative care focuses specifically on relieving pain and discomfort. Its purpose is to help people suffering so they may better enjoy life and is not limited to the dying.

Comfort care is, as the name implies, all about comfort. It usually begins with a medical recommendation to shift goals from treatment to comfort because aggressive therapies aren't working. In this sense, it recognizes that end-of-life is approaching and modern medicine cannot cure the underlying causes or manage their symptoms. It does not mean that death is imminent.

Hospice care is for people who are actively dying. Some treatments like oxygen and medications to manage symptoms may continue, but hospice often brings increased attention from nurses, doctors, social workers, and chaplains. Hospice is frequently provided at home or in medical or residential care facilities. Importantly for families in the United States, hospice services are covered by Medicare.

Let's introduce *curative care* to better distinguish between the three end-of-life care forms. Such care aims to cure the patient or successfully manage their symptoms. Palliative care may accompany it when a patient has discomfort or is in pain.

Throughout a journey with dementia, your loved one may receive palliative care, comfort care, and hospice care. In some cases, patients may go on and off of any of these forms of care if they show improvement. I've seen people go into comfort care and experience substantial improvement in their symptoms with new medication management. I've also witnessed people go on hospice and improve sufficiently to qualify no longer.

Responding

Most often, people caring for loved ones with Alzheimer's or dementia are fully involved with medical professionals. If your loved one shows any alarming changes, including a loss of appetite, weight loss, lethargy, stopping walking, or losing their will to live, contact their medical professional immediately. None of the three forms of care addressed here begin without first evaluating curative options.

What we caregivers must do is prepare. Many families choose to execute an estate plan or trust. This legal document can simplify settling your loved one's estate after passing. The trust will likely include Durable Power(s) of Attorney and Healthcare Power(s) of Attorney with Advance Directive(s), or ADs. The AD will describe the desired medical treatment level for several scenarios. It may also include expectations related to treatment when dementia is present, including choosing comfort care or a Do Not Resuscitate clause (DNR).

Notably, a person with diagnosed dementia can't legally execute a trust due to their mental impairment. Families must complete these documents while their loved ones may sign them. Be sure to use a reputable attorney specializing in trusts and estate planning.

As described in the chapter on **Caregiver Guilt**, a Physician's Orders for Life-Sustaining Treatment, or POLST, are medical directives for patients with advanced illnesses that limit treatment. The document is created collaboratively between a physician, the patient, the person holding power of attorney over the patient's health, and sometimes the patient's family. If warranted, discuss a POLST with your loved one's physician.

Closing Thoughts

Throughout this book, I've tried to describe some of the most common behaviors and situations family members face when caring for their loved ones with dementia. Most persons with dementia will exhibit some behaviors, not all, so I wanted to include the most challenging. I hope you never face the most difficult among them but that our discussions are helpful for those you do face.

Most people will recognize at least some of the situations we addressed. My advice for each can help guide your approach, especially the highlighted pitfalls to avoid.

I wanted to leave family caregivers some final thoughts and encouragement for your journey.

Be Compassionate to Yourself

After more than fifteen years of specializing in dementia care, I know that most family caregivers are too hard on themselves. They often feel they should have done more or something different. They question their ability and decisions and worry that others will judge them unfairly. I refer all caregivers to review the chapter on **Caregiver Guilt**.

Give up the guilt! You are likely facing new situations caring for a loved one who may have cared for you. You're going to make mistakes, and you're going to have some conflict with your loved one, other family members, and even acquaintances, even as you try to do your best. You're also facing new paperwork and new medical, legal, and financial situations you may never face again. Only professionals working with many people with dementia for years have wisdom and experience in this area. Learn from mistakes, grow from experiences, and cut yourself slack.

TALK WITH OTHERS AND SEEK ADVICE

Too many caregivers try to use instinct and experience as a guide to the new situation with their loved ones. Professionals will dispense good advice, but it goes only so far.

Know that every situation and challenge you face has been previously faced by someone else. Talk to others about your situation and be open to good advice. As mentioned several times throughout this book, support groups are safe places for caregivers to share experiences and seek advice from others. Look for support groups in your area and make a point of attending regularly. If you can't find an in-person group in your area, turn to the Internet for an online option. The important thing is to share your experiences and to learn from others.

GET HELP

Remember that you do not need to do everything yourself, and you don't have to learn every lesson the hard way through trial and error. Much information can be found online, but exercise caution because several for-profit companies offer free resources and advice after registering or providing details of your case. These offers may seem innocent, but companies that pay to land in your search results have a financial motive. Instead, look for information from government sources or not-for-profit medical organizations.

Depending on your resources, consider hiring a professional care manager who specializes in dementia care. If that's not an option, look for community-based support from local places of worship, senior centers, and local hospitals or health organizations.

Caring for someone with dementia is an obligation, but it needn't be all-consuming in most cases. With the proper support, you can continue to lead an enjoyable life!

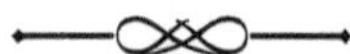

Online Resources from Lauren Mahakian

Lauren offers dementia care management services both in person and by telephone. She also holds a Memory, Coffee, and Compassion Support Group for dementia caregivers, both in-person and online.

Care Management
familyconnectmemorycare.com/services/care-management

Support Groups
familyconnectmemorycare.com/support-groups

More Information
info@familyconnectcare.com

www.ingramcontent.com/pod-product-compliance
Lightning Source LLC
Chambersburg PA
CBHW050919260726
48660CB00001B/283